T0276640

Quality Control

Quality Control

Edited by Theresa Hoon

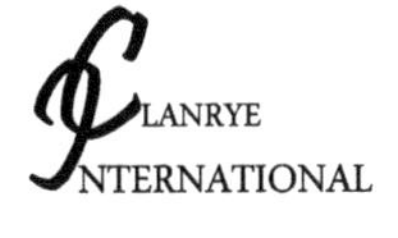

New Jersey

Published by Clanrye International,
55 Van Reypen Street,
Jersey City, NJ 07306, USA
www.clanryeinternational.com

Quality Control
Edited by Theresa Heen

International Standard Book Number: 978-1-63240-434-3 (Hardback)

Printed in the United States of America.

Contents

Preface

This book was inspired by the evolution of our times, to answer the curiosity of inquisitive minds. Many developments have occurred across the globe in the recent past which has transformed the progress in the field.

Quality control is a procedure or set of procedures formulated for the purpose of maintaining standards in manufactured products. This book presents a comprehensive overview of the important elements of quality control. It gives a contemporary account of methods used to design quality models. It is created to be used as a text for courses on quality control for students of industrial engineering at the advanced and undergraduate level. The book can also serve as a reference for researchers in related areas looking for a synopsis of the main concepts of quality control.

This book was developed from a mere concept to drafts to chapters and finally compiled together as a complete text to benefit the readers across all nations. To ensure the quality of the content we instilled two significant steps in our procedure. The first was to appoint an editorial team that would verify the data and statistics provided in the book and also select the most appropriate and valuable contributions from the plentiful contributions we received from authors worldwide. The next step was to appoint an expert of the topic as the Editor-in-Chief, who would head the project and finally make the necessary amendments and modifications to make the text reader-friendly. I was then commissioned to examine all the material to present the topics in the most comprehensible and productive format.

I would like to take this opportunity to thank all the contributing authors who were supportive enough to contribute their time and knowledge to this project. I also wish to convey my regards to my family who have been extremely supportive during the entire project.

Editor

Section 1

Statistical Quality Control

Chapter 1

Toward a Better Quality Control of Weather Data

Kenneth Hubbard, Jinsheng You and
[illegible]

Additional information is available at the end of the chapter

1. Introduction

Previous studies have documented various QC tools for use with weather data (26; 4; 6; 25; 9; 3; 10; 16; 18). As a result, there has been good progress in the automated QC ofweather indices, especially the daily maximum/ minimum air temperature. The QC of precipitation is more difficult than for temperature; this is due to the fact that the spatial and temporal variability of a variable (2) is related to the confidence in identifying outliers. Another approach to maintaining quality of data is to conduct intercomparisons of redundant measurements taken at a site. For example, the designers of the United States Climate Reference Network (USCRN) made it possible to compare between redundant measurements by specifying a rain gauge with multiple vibrating wires in order to avoid a single point of failure in the measurement process. In this case the three vibrating wires can be compared to determine whether or not the outputs are comparable and any outlying values can result in a site visit. CRN also includes three temperature sensors at each site for the purpose of comparison.

Generally identifying outliers involves tests designed to work on data from a single site (9) or tests designed to compare a station's data against the data from neighboring stations (16). Statistical decisions play a large role in quality control efforts but, increasingly there are rules introduced which depend upon the physical system involved. Examples of these are the testing of hourly solar radiation against the clear sky envelope (Allen, 1996; Geiger, et al., 2002) and the use of soil heat diffusion theory to determine soil temperature validity (Hu, et al., 2002). It is now realized that quality assurance (QA) is best suited when made a seamless process between staff operating the quality control software at a centralized location where data is ingested and technicians responsible for maintenance of sensors in the field (16; 10).

Quality assurance software consists of procedures or rules against which data are tested. Each procedure will either accept the data as being true or reject the data and label it as an outlier. This hypothesis (Ho) testing of the data and the statistical decision to accept the data or to note it as an outlier can have the outcomes shown in Table 1:

Statistical Decision	True Situation	
	Ho True	Ho False
Accept Ho	No error	Type II error
Reject Ho	Type I error	No Error

Table 1. The classification of possible outcomes in testing of a quality assurance hypothesis.

Take the simple case of testing a variable against limits. If we take as our hypothesis that the data for a measured variable is valid only if it lies within ±3σ of the mean (X), then assuming a normal distribution we expect to accept Ho 99.73% of the time in the abscense of errors. The values that lie beyond X±3σ will be rejected and we will make a Type I error when we encounter valid values beyond these limits. In these cases, we are rejecting Ho when the value is actually valid and we therefore expect to make a Type I error 0.27% of the time assuming for this discussion that the data has no errant values. If we encounter a bad value inside the limits X±3σ we will accept it when it is actually false (the value is not valid) and this would lead to a Type II error. In this simple example, reducing the limits against which the data values are tested will produce more Type I errors and fewer Type II errors while increasing the limits leads to fewer Type I errors and more Type II errors. For quality assurance software, study is necessary to achieve a balance wherein one reduces the Type II errors (mark more "errant" data as having failed the test) while not increasing Type I errors to the point where valid extremes are brought into question. Because Type I errors cannot be avoided, it is prudent for data managers to always keep the original measured values regardless of the quality testing results and offer users an input into specifying the limits $\pm f\sigma$ beyond which the data will be marked as potential outliers.

In this chapter we point to three major contributions. The first is the explicit treatment of Type I and Type II errors in the evaluation of the performance of quality control procedures to provide a basis for comparison of procedures. The second is to illustrate how the selection of parameters in the quality control process can be tailored to individual needs in regions or sub-regions of a wide-spread network. Finally, we introduce a new spatial regression test (SRT) which uses a subset of the neighboring stations to provide the "best fit" to the target station. This spatial regression weighted procedure produces non-biased estimates with characteristics which make it possible to specify statistical confidence intervals for testing data at the target station.

2. A Dataset with seeded errors

A dataset consisting of original data and seeded errors (18) is used to evaluate the performance of the different QC approaches for temperature and precipitation. The QC procedures can be tracked to determine the number of seeded errors that are identified. The ratio of errors identified by a QC procedure to the total number of errors seeded is a metric that can be compared across the range of error magnitudes introduced. The data used to create the seeded error dataset was from the U.S. Cooperative Observer Network as archived in the National Climatic Data Center (NCDC).We used the Applied Climate Information (ACIS) system to access stations with daily data available for all months from 1971~2000(see 24). The data have been assessed using NCDC procedures and are referred to as "clean" data. Note, however, that "clean" does not necessarily infer that the data are true values but, means instead that the largest outliers have been removed.

About 2% of all observations were selected on a random basis to be seeded with an error. The magnitude of the error was also determined in a random manner. A random number, *r*, was selected using a random number generator operating on a uniform distribution with a mean of zero and range of ±3.5. This number was then multiplied by the standard deviation (σ_x) of the variable in question to obtain the error magnitude *E* for the randomly selected observation *x*:

$$E_x = \sigma_x r \tag{1}$$

The variable*r* is not used when the error would produce negative precipitation, (E_x+*x*)<0., Thus the seeded error value is skewed distributed when *r*<0 but roughly uniformly distributed when *r*> 0. The selection of 3.5 for the range is arbitrary but does serve to produce a large range of errors (±3.5σ_x).This approach to producing a seeded data set is used below in some of the comparisons.

3. The spatial regression test (estimates)and Inverse Distance Weighted Estimates (IDW)

When checking data from a site, missing values are sometimes present. For modeling and other purposes where continuous data are required, an estimate is needed for the missing value. We will refer to the station which is missing the data as the target station. The IDW method has been used to make estimates (x') at the target stations from surrounding observations (x_i).

$$x' = \sum_{i=1}^{N} (x_i / f(d_i)) \ / \sum_{i=1}^{N} 1 / f(d_i) \tag{2}$$

Where d_i is the distance from the target station to each of the nearby stations, f(di) is a function relying on d_i(in our case we took $f(d_i)=1/d_i$). This approach assumes that the nearest stations will be most representative of the target site.

Spatial Regression (SRT) is a new method that provides an estimate for the target station and can be used to check that the observation (when not missing) falls inside the confidence interval formed from N estimates based on N "best fits" between the target station and neighboring stations during a time period of length n. The surrounding stations are selected be specifying a radius around the station and finding those stations with the closest statistical agreement to the target station. Additional requirements for station selection are that the variable to be tested is one of the variables measured at the target site and the data for that variable spans the data period to be tested. A station that otherwise qualifies could also be eliminated from consideration if more than half of the data is missing for the time span (e.g. more than 12 missing dayswhere n=24) First non-biased, preliminary estimates x_{lt} are derived by use ofthe coefficients derived from linear regression, so for any time t, and for each surrounding station (y_{lt}) an estimate is formed.

$$x_i^{'} = a_i + b_i y_i \tag{3}$$

The approach obtains an un-biased estimate (x') by utilizing the standard error of estimate (s) for each of the linear regressions in the weighting process.

$$x' = \sum_{i=1}^{N} (x_i^{'} / s_i^2) / \sum_{i=1}^{N} 1 / s_i^2 \tag{4}$$

$$N / s'^2 = \sum_{i=1}^{N} 1 / s_i^2 \tag{5}$$

The surrounding stations are ranked according to the magnitude of the standard error of estimate and the N stations with the lowest s values are used in the weighting process:

This approach provides more weight to the stations that are the best estimators of the target station. Because the stations used in (4) are a subset of the neighboring stations the estimate is not an areal average but a spatial regression weighted estimate

The approach differs from inverse distance weighting in that the standard error of estimate has a statistical distribution, therefore confidence intervals can be calculated on the basis of s' and the station value (x) can be tested to determine whether or not it falls within the *confidence* intervals.

$$x' - fs' \leq x \leq x' + fs' \tag{6}$$

If the above relationship holds, then the datum passes the spatial test. This relationship indicates that with successively larger values of f, the number of potential Type I errors decreases. Unlike distance weighting techniques, this approach does not assume that the best station to compare against is the closest station but, instead looks to the relationships between the actual station data to settle which stations should be used to make the estimates and what weighting these stations should receive. An example of the estimates obtained from the SRT is given in Table 2.

ating yi based on x			20E 35S	Havelock	82E 20S	12W 55N	51E 13S							
A254739	A254749	days	x	y1	y2	y3	y4	x'1	x'2	x'3	x'4	x'1/s1'^2	x'2/s2'^2	x'3/s3'^2
83.696	85.586	6/1/2011	85.1	85.5	83.4	83.7	85.6	85.51	84.30	84.82	84.62	47.016	92.680	170.315
85.004	87.584	6/2/2011	86.2	86.2	85.3	85.6	87.6	86.28	86.33	86.78	86.62	47.438	94.906	174.255
89.942	92.282	6/3/2011	91.9	89.5	90.0	89.9	92.3	89.73	91.33	91.24	91.30	49.338	100.408	183.214
85.478	85.1	6/4/2011	84.1	85.9	83.5	85.5	95.1	85.91	84.42	86.65	84.14	47.238	92.806	173.995
[illegible]	[illegible]	6/5/2011	96.3	94.9	94.1	94.5	97.3	95.49	95.67	95.89	[illegible]	[illegible]	105.175	192.545
[illegible]	[illegible]	6/6/2011	99.0	[illegible]	[illegible]	97.6	101.0	98.83	99.51	99.09	99.99	54.341	109.395	198.977
95.918	[illegible]	[illegible]	[illegible]	[illegible]	[illegible]	[illegible]	[illegible]	[illegible]	[illegible]	[illegible]	97.73	53.349	107.841	195.557
83.066	86.288	6/8/2011	[illegible]	[illegible]	[illegible]	[illegible]	[illegible]	[illegible]	[illegible]	[illegible]	[illegible]	[illegible]	[illegible]	[illegible]
69.674	72.878	6/9/2011	71.0	71.8	71.9	69.7	[illegible]	[illegible]	[illegible]	[illegible]	[illegible]	[illegible]	[illegible]	[illegible]
66.2	67.766	6/10/2011	66.2	69.8	67.6	66.2	67.8	68.77	67.59	66.82	66.86	[illegible]	[illegible]	[illegible]
75.758	76.694	6/11/2011	76.2	76.2	74.8	75.8	76.7	75.53	75.19	76.65	75.76	41.527	82.663	153.921
77.324	78.98	6/12/2011	78.8	77.9	77.7	77.3	79.0	77.43	78.29	78.26	78.04	42.572	86.065	157.155
69.314	70.97	6/13/2011	69.2	70.3	69.9	69.3	71.0	69.23	69.98	70.03	70.05	38.066	76.930	140.612
76.028	78.728	6/14/2011	78.1	79.5	78.1	76.0	78.7	79.12	78.67	76.93	77.79	43.501	86.485	154.478
84.632	86.396	6/15/2011	86.4	85.0	85.3	84.6	86.4	84.97	86.35	85.78	85.43	46.720	94.927	172.248
85.118	86.27	6/16/2011	86.8	85.3	84.0	85.1	86.3	85.24	84.94	86.28	85.31	46.868	93.373	173.252
90.266	92.732	6/17/2011	91.3	92.5	90.9	90.3	92.7	92.92	92.33	91.58	91.75	51.090	101.500	183.884
80.312	82.904	6/18/2011	81.5	82.9	81.4	80.3	82.9	82.71	82.22	81.34	81.95	45.475	90.391	163.326
85.118	87.458	6/19/2011	85.6	86.6	85.5	85.1	87.5	86.66	86.60	86.28	86.49	47.649	95.200	173.252
86.81	88.448	6/20/2011	87.9	88.2	86.7	86.8	88.4	88.35	87.88	88.02	87.48	48.578	96.607	176.746
71.258	72.788	6/21/2011	72.0	72.9	71.9	71.3	72.8	72.07	72.16	72.03	71.87	39.628	79.324	144.627
74.948	76.586	6/22/2011	76.7	75.0	74.4	74.9	76.6	74.26	74.83	75.82	75.65	40.831	82.264	152.248
76.604	78.62	6/23/2011	77.1	78.9	76.4	76.6	78.6	78.45	76.87	77.52	77.68	43.132	84.511	155.668
78.17	80.168	6/24/2011	79.4	79.4	78.3	78.2	80.2	78.96	78.92	79.13	79.22	43.417	86.758	158.902
80.564	82.544	6/25/2011	82.0	80.8	80.6	80.6	82.5	80.52	81.33	81.60	81.59	44.272	89.404	163.846
81.302	82.814	6/26/2011	82.1	82.3	82.1	81.3	82.8	82.09	82.91	82.36	81.86	45.137	91.147	165.370
78.044	80.06	6/27/2011	79.1	79.8	77.9	78.0	80.1	79.37	78.54	79.00	79.12	43.638	86.338	158.642
79.61	81.716	6/28/2011	81.1	80.2	79.1	79.6	81.7	79.87	79.80	80.62	80.77	43.913	87.724	161.876
89.78	91.76	6/29/2011	91.3	89.7	89.3	89.8	91.8	89.96	90.55	91.08	90.78	49.465	99.547	182.880
98.78	101.48	6/30/2011	100.0	100.3	98.4	98.8	101.5	101.25	100.29	100.33	100.47	55.671	110.256	201.467

Linear regression parameters						sum(1/si^2)	s'
	Slope	1.066	1.061	1.029	0.997		
	Intercept	-5.687	-4.170	-1.265	-0.705	5.73249	0.83533
	Si(x,yi)	1.349	0.954	0.706	0.694		

0.069812	0.208934							
0.382169	0.206952							
0.48731	0.408523	One example for day 30 (i=1 to 4 for four reference stations) :						
6.273045	3.18E-05	yi	1.1	0.4	-0.7	-0.6	1.43312	0.83533

Table 2 An example of QC using Spatial Regression Test (SRT) method for daily maximum temperature estimation (unit: F). Stations are from the Automated Weather Data Network and locations are on an East-West by North South street naming convention. The original station (Lincoln 20E 35S) is labeled x while the four neighboring stations are y1,y2, y3, and y4. Equation 3 is used to derive the unbiased estimates $x_1^{'}$, $x_2^{'}$ etc. for n=30. The final estimate x(est) is determined from the unbiased estimates using equations 4 and 5.

Using the above methodology, the rate of error detection can be pre-selected. The reader should note that the results are presented in terms of the fraction of data flagged against the range of f values (defined above) rather than selecting one f value on an arbitrary basis. This type of analysis makes it possible to select the specific f values for stations in differing climate regimes that would keep the Type I error rate uniform across the country. For example for sake of illustration, suppose the goal is to select f values which keep the potential Type I errors to about two percent. A representative set of stations and years can be pre-analyzed prior to QC to determine the f values appropriate to achieve this goal.The SRT method implicitly resolves the bias between variables at different stations induced by elevation difference or other attributes.

Tables 2 and 3 show the use of SRT (equations 3, 4 and 5 above). The data in the example are retrieved from the AWDN stations for the month of June 2011. Only one month was used in this example. The stations are located in the city of Lincoln, NE, USA. The station being tested is Lincoln 20E 35S and is labeled x while the neighboring stations are labeled y1, y2, y3, and y4. The slope (ai), interception (bi), and standard errors of the linear regression between the x and yi are computed. The non-biased estimation of x from data at neighboring stations (yi) are shown as x'1, x'2, x'3, and x'4. The values normalized s by the standard errors ($x'i/si^2$) are used in equation 4 to create the estimation x(est). The last column shows the bias between the true X value and the estimated value (x(est)) from the four stations. We see that the sum of bias of the 30 days has a value of 0.00, which is expected because the estimates using the SRT method are un-biased. The standard error of this regression estimation is 0.83 F. Here, for instance, where f was chosen as 3, any value that is smaller than -2.5 F or larger than 2.5 F will be treated as an outlier. In this example no value of x-x(est) was marked as an outlier.

	Original data at Stations, Lincoln NE, USA					estimated x from y				Normalized by s'					
	20E 35S	Havelock	82E 20S	12W 55N	51E 13S										
days	x	y1	y2	y3	y4	x'1	x'2	x'3	x'4	x'1/s1'^2	x'2/s2'^2	x'3/s3'^2	x'4/s4'^2	X(est)	x-x(est)
6/1/2011	85.1	85.5	83.4	83.7	85.6	85.64	84.39	84.84	84.66	54.055	98.238	164.200	171.671	84.8	-0.31
6/2/2011	86.2	86.2	85.3	85.6	87.6	86.39	86.39	86.80	86.64	54.533	100.577	167.980	175.693	86.6	0.46
6/3/2011	91.9	89.5	90.0	89.9	92.3	89.80	91.36	91.24	91.31	56.686	106.360	176.575	185.152	91.1	-0.81
6/4/2011	84.1	85.9	83.5	85.5	85.1	86.03	84.50	86.67	84.18	54.306	98.370	167.731	170.692	85.3	1.14
6/5/2011	96.3	94.9	94.1	94.5	97.3	95.49	95.67	95.86	96.28	60.274	111.370	185.527	195.227	95.9	-0.35
6/6/2011	99.8	98.0	97.7	97.6	101.0	98.79	99.48	99.05	99.96	62.356	115.806	191.697	202.692	99.4	-0.32
6/7/2011	97.2	96.3	96.4	95.9	98.7	97.00	98.07	97.36	97.71	61.231	114.173	188.416	198.126	97.6	0.35
6/8/2011	83.5	86.4	84.8	83.1	86.3	86.53	85.88	84.20	85.36	54.617	99.981	162.951	173.084	85.2	1.69
6/9/2011	71.0	71.8	71.9	69.7	72.9	71.23	72.35	70.49	72.04	44.964	84.223	136.417	146.085	71.5	0.47
6/10/2011		69.8	67.6	66.2	67.8	69.11	67.80	66.93	66.97	43.624	78.926	129.534	135.792	67.4	
6/11/2011	76.2	76.2	74.8	75.8	76.7	75.78	75.34	76.72	75.83	47.835	87.710	148.472	153.768	76.0	-0.15
6/12/2011	78.8	77.9	77.7	77.3	79.0	77.66	78.41	78.32	78.10	49.019	91.285	151.575	158.370	78.2	-0.65
6/13/2011	69.2	70.3	69.9	69.3	71.0	69.57	70.17	70.12	70.15	43.911	81.685	135.704	142.243	70.1	0.85
6/14/2011	78.1	79.5	78.1	76.0	78.7	79.32	78.79	76.99	77.85	50.071	91.727	149.007	157.863	77.9	-0.20
6/15/2011	86.4	85.0	85.3	84.6	86.4	85.10	86.41	85.80	85.46	53.720	100.599	166.054	173.301	85.7	-0.67
6/16/2011	86.8	85.3	84.0	85.1	86.3	85.37	85.01	86.30	85.34	53.887	98.966	167.017	173.048	85.6	-1.18
6/17/2011		92.5	90.9	90.3	92.7	92.95	92.35	91.57	91.75	58.672	107.508	177.217	186.058	91.9	
6/18/2011	81.5	82.9	81.4	80.3	82.9	82.87	82.32	81.38	82.00	52.308	95.832	157.495	166.271	81.9	0.47
6/19/2011	85.6	86.6	85.5	85.1	87.5	86.77	86.66	86.30	86.52	54.772	100.886	167.017	175.440	86.5	0.93
6/20/2011	87.9	88.2	86.7	86.8	88.4	88.44	87.93	88.03	87.50	55.825	102.365	170.370	177.433	87.9	0.01
6/21/2011	72.0	72.9	71.9	71.3	72.8	72.37	72.33	72.11	71.95	45.682	84.201	139.556	145.904	72.1	0.13
6/22/2011	76.7	75.0	74.4	74.9	76.6	74.53	74.98	75.89	75.72	47.045	87.291	146.867	153.550	75.5	-1.18
6/23/2011	77.1	78.9	76.4	76.6	78.6	78.66	77.01	77.58	77.74	49.653	89.652	150.148	157.645	77.6	0.50
6/24/2011	79.4	79.4	78.3	78.2	80.2	79.17	79.04	79.19	79.28	49.976	92.014	153.251	160.762	79.2	-0.24
6/25/2011	82.0	80.8	80.6	80.6	82.5	80.71	81.43	81.64	81.64	50.945	94.795	157.994	165.546	81.5	-0.46
6/26/2011	82.1	82.3	82.1	81.3	82.8	82.26	83.00	82.39	81.91	51.925	96.627	159.456	166.089	82.3	0.24
6/27/2011	79.1	79.8	77.9	78.0	80.1	79.57	78.66	79.06	79.17	50.227	91.572	153.001	160.545	79.1	0.00
6/28/2011	81.1	80.2	79.1	79.6	81.7	80.06	79.91	80.66	80.82	50.538	93.029	156.104	163.879	80.5	-0.61
6/29/2011	91.3	89.7	89.3	89.8	91.8	90.03	90.58	91.07	90.79	56.830	105.455	176.254	184.101	90.8	-0.57
6/30/2011	100.0	100.3	98.4	98.8	101.5	101.17	100.25	100.29	100.44	63.863	116.711	194.087	203.671	100.4	0.45
	Slope	1.053	1.053	1.024	0.993										0.00

Table 3 An example of estimating missing data Spatial Regression Test (SRT) method for daily maximum temperature estimation (unit: F). In this example, two days were assumed missing: 6/10 and 6/17 and were estimated using equations 3, 4, and 5 (see highlighted values in the x(est) column. Stations are from the Automated Weather Data Network and locations are on an East-West by North South naming convention. The original station (Lincoln 20E 35S) is labeled x while the four neighboring stations are y1,y2, y3, and y4. Equation 3 is used to derive the unbiased estimates x_1', x_2' etc. for n=28. The final estimate x(est) is determined from the unbiased estimates using equations 4 and 5.

If one value or several values at the station x is missing, the x(est) will provide an estimate for the missing data entry (see Table 3). The example in Table 3 shows that the value of x is missing in June 10 and June 17, 2011, through the SRT method we can obtain the estimates as 67.4 F and 91.9 F for the two days independent of the true values of 66.2 F and 91.3 F with a bias of 1.2 F and 0.6 F, respectively. Here we note that the estimated values of the two days are slightly different than those estimated in Table 2 because there are 2 less values to include in the regression.

4. Providing estimates: robustness of SRT method and weakness of IDW method

The SRT method was tested against the Inverse Distance Weighted (IDW) method to determine the representativeness of estimates obtained (29). The SRT method outperformed the IDW method in complex terrain and complex microclimates. To illustrate this we have taken the data from a national cooperative observer site at Silver Lake Brighton, UT.The elevation at Silver Lake Brighton is 8740 ft. The nearest neighboring station is located at Soldier Summit at an elevation of 7486 ft. This data is for the year 2002. Daily estimates for maximum and minimum temperature were obtained for each day by temporarily removing the observation from that day and applying both the IDW (eq. 1) and the SRT (eq.2) methodsagainst 15 neighboring stations. The estimations for the SRT method were derived by applying the method (deriving the un-biased estimates) every 24 data.

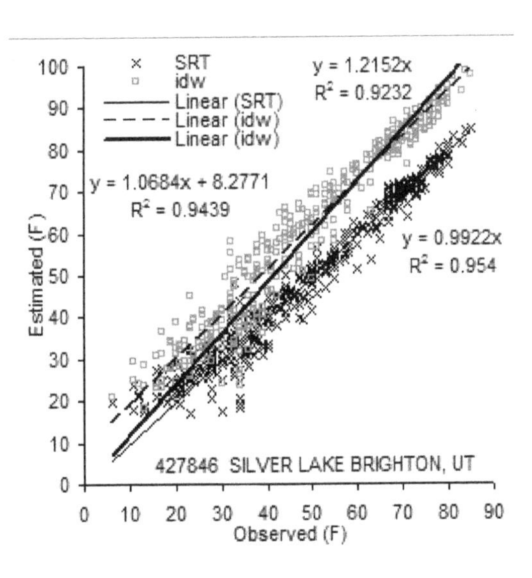

Figure 1. The results of estimating maximum temperature at Silver Lake Brighton, UT for both the IDW and the SRT methods.

Fig. 1 shows the result for maximum temperature at Silver Lake Brighton, Utah. The IDW approach results in a large bias. The best fit line for IDW indicates the estimates are systematically high by over 8 F (8.27); the slope is also greater than one (1.0684). When the best fit line for IDW estimates was forced through zero, the slope was 1.2152. On the other hand the estimates from the SRT indicate almost no bias as evidenced by the best-fit slope (0.9922).

For the minimum temperature estimates a similar result was found (Fig. 2). The slope of the best-fit line for the SRT indicates an unbiased (0.9931) while the slope for the IDW estimates indicates a large bias on the order of 20% (slope = 1.1933). The reader should note the SRT unbiased estimators are derived every 24 days (see) and that applying the SRT only once for the entire period will degrade the results shown (7).

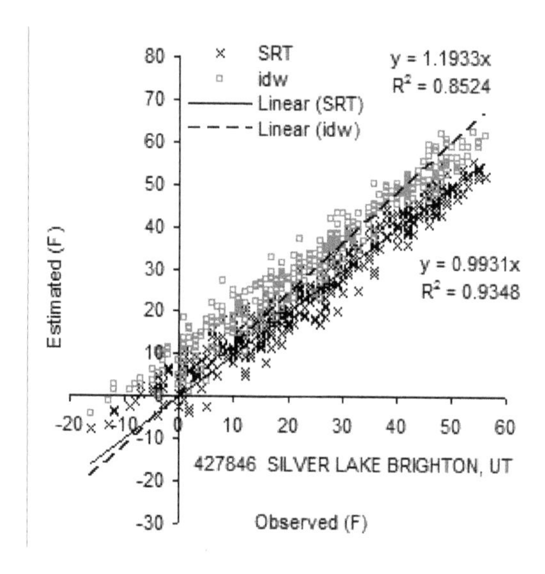

Figure 2. The results of estimating minimum temperature at Silver Lake Brighton, UT for both the IDW and the SRT methods.

5. Techniques used to improve the quality control procedures during the extreme events.

Quality of data during the extreme events such as strong cold fronts and hurricanes may decrease resulting in a higher number of "true" outliers than that during the normal climate conditions. (28) carefully analyzed the sample examples of these extreme weather conditions to quantitatively demonstrate the causes of the outliers and then developed tools to reset the Type II error flags. The following discussion will elaborate on this technique.

5.1. Relationship between interval of measurement and QA failures

Analyses were conducted to prepare artificial max and min temperature records (not the measurements, but the values identified as the max and min from the hourly time series) for different times-of-observation from available hourly time series of measurements. The observation time for coop weather stations varies from site-to-site. Here we define the AM station, PM station, and nighttime station according to the time of observation (i.e. morning, afternoon-evening, and midnight respectively). The cooperative network has a higher number of PM stations but AM measurements are also common; the Automated Weather Data Network uses a midnight to midnight observation period.

The daily precipitation accumulates the precipitation for the past 24 hours ending at the time of observation. The precipitation during the time interval may not match the precipitation from nearby neighboring stations due to event slicing, i.e. precipitation may occur both before and after a station's time of observation. Thus, a single storm can be sliced into two observation periods.

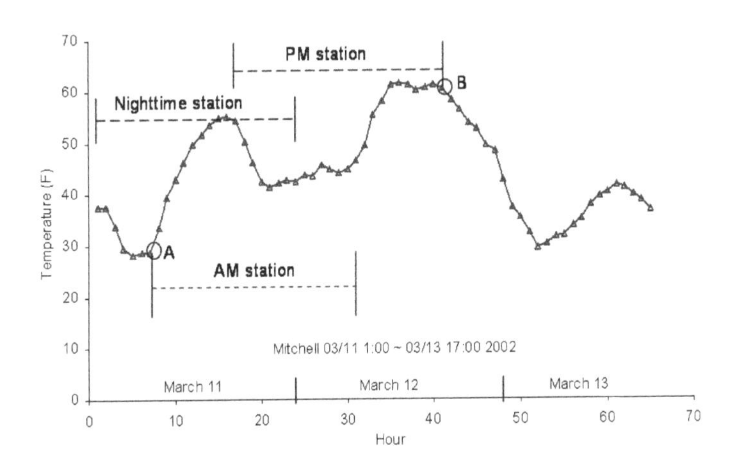

Figure 3. Example time intervals for observations at Mitchell, NE (after 28).

The measurements of the maximum and the minimum temperature are the result of making discrete intervals on a continuous variable. The maximum or minimum temperature takes the maximum value or the minimum value of temperature during the specific time interval. Thus the maximum temperature or the minimum temperature is not necessarily the maximum or minimum value of a diurnal cycle. Examples of the differences were obtained from three time intervals (see Fig 3) after28)). The hourly measurements of air temperature were retrieved from 1:00 March 11 to 17:00 March 13, 2002 at Mitchell, NE. The times of observation are marked. Point *A* shows the minimum air temperature obtained for March 11 for AM stations, and *B* is the maximum temperature obtained for March 13 at the PM stations. The minimum temperature may carry over to the following interval for AM stations and the maximum temperature may carry over to the following interval for PM stations. We have therefore marked these as problematic in Table 4to note that the thermodynamic state of the atmosphere will be represented differently for AM and PM stations. Through analysis of the time series of AM, PM and midnight calculated from the high quality hourly data we find that measurements obtained at the PM station have a higher risk of QA failure when compared to neighboring AM stations. The difference in temperature at different observation times may reach 20 °F for temperature and several inches for precipitation. Therefore the QA failures may not be due to sensor problems but, to comparing data from stations where the sensors are employed differently. To avoid this problem AM stations can be compared to AM stations, PM stations to PM stations, etc. Note this problem will be solved if modernization of network provides hourly or sub-hourly data at most station sites.

	AM station	PM station	Nighttime station (AWDN)
Time intervals (e.g.)	~7:00	~ 17:00	~midnight
Maximum temperature		Problematic	
Minimum temperature	Problematic		
Precipitation	Good	Good	Good

Table 4. Time interval and possible performance of three intervals of measurements.

5.2. 1993 floods

Quality control procedures were applied to the data for the 1993 Midwest floods over the Missouri River Basin and part of the upper Mississippi River Basin, where heavy rainfall and floods occurred (28). The spatial regression test performs well and flags 5~7 % of the data for most of the area at f=3. The spatial patterns of the fraction of the flagged records do not coincide with the spatial pattern of return period. For example, the southeast part of Nebraska does not show a high fraction of flagged records although most stations have return periods of more than 1000 years. While, upper Wisconsin has a higher fraction of flagged records although the precipitation for this case has a lower return period in that area.

The analysis shows a significantly higher fraction of flagged records using AWDN stations in North Dakota than in other states. This demonstrates that the differences in daily precipitation obtained from stations with different times of observation contributed to the high fraction of QA failures. A high risk of failure would occur in such cases when the measurements of the current station and the reference station are obtained from PM stations and AM stations respectively. The situation worsens if the measurements at weather stations were obtained from different time intervals and the distribution of stations with different time-of-observation is unfavorable. This would be the case for an isolated AM or PM station.

Among the 13 flags at Grand Forks, 9 flags may be due to the different times of observation or perhaps the size and spacing of clouds (28). Four other flags occurred during localized precipitation events, in which only a single station received significant precipitation. Higher precipitation entries occurring in isolation are more likely to be identified as potential outliers. These problems were expected to be avoided by examining the precipitation over larger intervals, e.g. summing consecutive days into event totals.

5.3. 2002 drought events

No significant relationship is found between the topography and the fraction of flagged records. Some clusters of stations with high flag frequency are located along the mountains; however, other mountainous stations do not show this pattern. Moreover, some locations with similar topography have different patterns. For the State of Colorado, a high fraction of flags occurs along the foothills of the Rocky Mountains where the mountains meet the high plains. A high fraction was also found along interstate highways 25 and 70 in east Colorado. These situations may come about because the weather stations were managed by different organizations or different sensors were employed at these stations. These differences lead to possible higher fraction of flagged records in some areas.

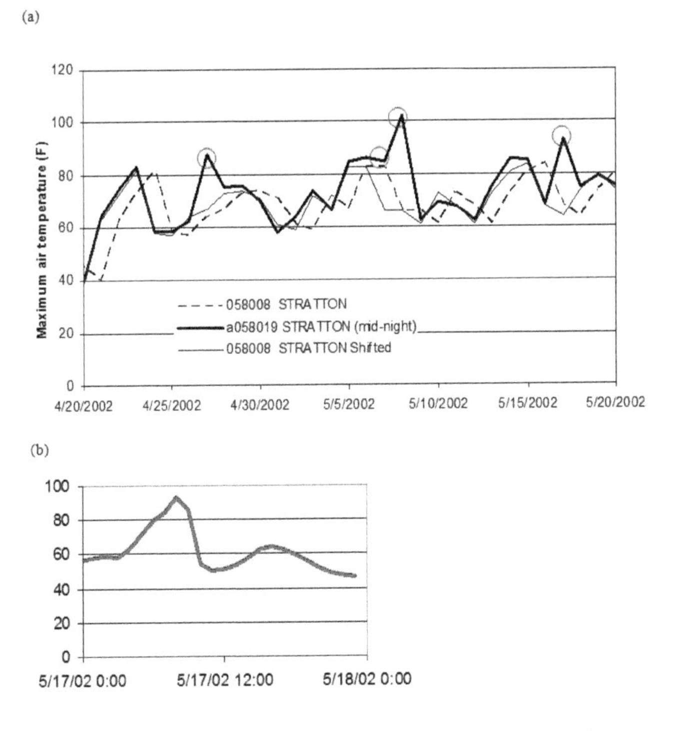

Figure 4. Time series of Stratton and a neighboring station during 2002 droughts. a) The daily time series of Tmax for Stratton and Stratton AWDN station (a058019). b) Hourly time series at Stratton AWDN station. (after 28).

Instrumental failures and abnormal events also lead to QA failures. Fig. 4 shows the time series of the Stratton Station in Color adooperated as part of the automated weather network. This station has nighttime (midnight) readings while all of the neighboring sites are AM or PM stations. Stratton thus has the most flagged records in the state (6): the highlighted records in Fig. 4 were flagged. We checked the hourly data time series to investigate the QA failure in the daily maximum temperature time series for the time period from April 20 to May 20, 2002. No value was found to support a Tmax of 88 for May 6 in the hourly time series, thus 88 °F appears to be an outlier. On May 7 a high of 85 °F is recorded for the PM station observation interval, in which the value of the afternoon of May 6 is recorded as the high on May 7. The 102 °F observation of May 8 at 6:00 AM appears to be an observation error caused by a spike in the instrument reading. The observation of 93 °F at 8:00 AM May 17 is supported by the hourly observation time series (see Fig. 4 (b)) and is apparently associated with a down burst from a decaying thunderstorm.

5.4. 1992 Andrew Hurricane

In Fig. 5 the evolution of the spatial pattern of flagged records from August 25 to August 28, 1992 during Hurricane Andrew and the corresponding daily weather maps shows a heavy pattern of flagging.. The flags in the spatial pattern figures are cumulative for the days indicated. The test shows that the spatial regression test explicitly marks the track of the tropical storm. Starting from the second land-fall of Hurricane Andrew at mid-south Louisiana, the weather stations along the route have flagged records. The wind field formed by Hurricane Andrew helps to define the influence zone of the hurricane on flags. Many stations without flags have daily precipitation of more than 2 inches as the hurricane passes, which confirms that the spatial regression test is performing reasonably well in the presence of high precipitation events.

5.5. Cold front in 1990

Flags for the cold front event during October, 1990 were examined. The maximum air temperature dropped by as much as 40 °F during the passage of the cold front. Spatial patterns of flags on October 6 coincide with the area traversed by the cold front and many stations were flagged in such states as North Dakota, South Dakota, Iowa, and Nebraska. On October 7, the cold front moved to southeast regions beyond Nebraska and Iowa. Of course nearby stations on opposite sides of the cold front may experience different temperatures thus leading to flags. This may be further complicated when different times of observation are involved. The cold front continues moving and the area of high frequency of flags also moves with the front correspondingly.

A similar phenomenon can be found in the test of the precipitation and the minimum temperature. A spatial regression test of any of these three variables can roughly mark the movements of the cold front events. The identified movements of the cold fronts and associated flagging of "good records" may lead to more manual work to examine the records. Simple pattern recognition tools have been developed to identify the spatial patterns of these flags and reset these flags automatically (see Fig. 6).

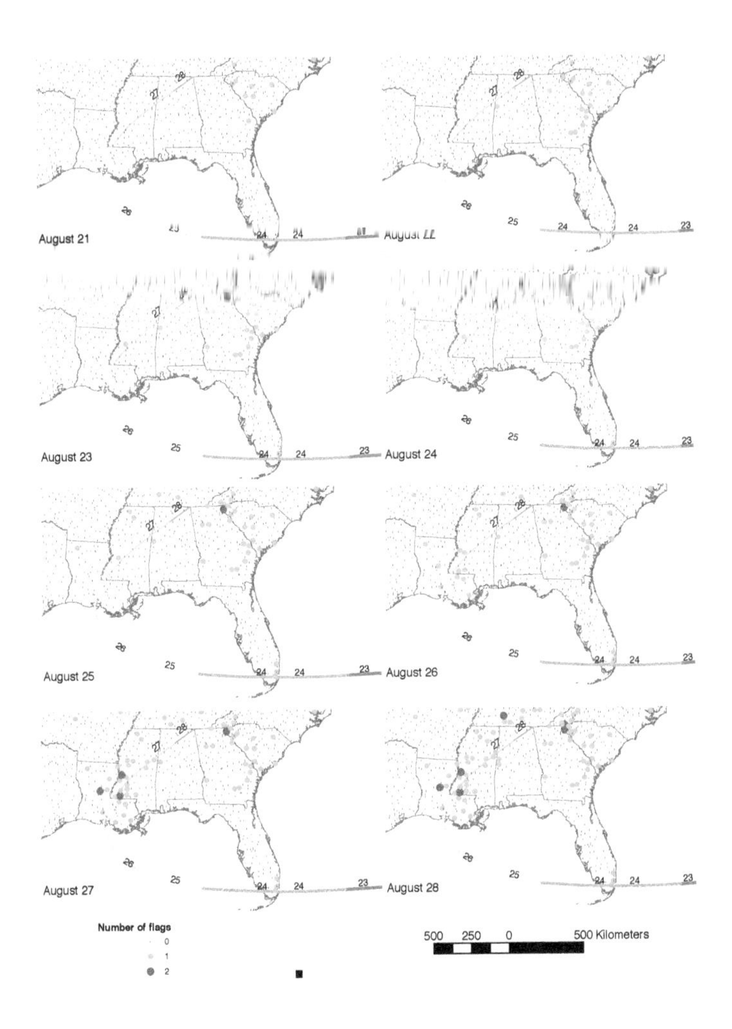

Figure 5. Daily weather maps and spatial pattern of flagged records for 1992 Andrew Hurricane events. (after 28).

The spatial patterns of flagged records are significant for both the spatial regression test of the cold front events and the tropical storm events. However, most of these flagged records are type I errors, thus we tested a simple pattern recognition tool to assist in reducing these flags. Differences still exist between the distribution patterns of the flagged records for the cold front event and the tropical storm events due to the characteristics of cold front events and tropical storm events. These differences are:

- Cold fronts have wide influence zones where the passages of the cold fronts are wider and the large areas immediately behind the cold front may have a significant flagged fraction of weather stations. The influence zones of the tropical storms are smaller where only the stations along the storm route and the neighboring stations have flags.

- Cold fronts exert influences on both the air temperature and precipitation. The temperature differences between the regions immediately ahead of the cold fronts and regions behind can reach 10~20 °C. The precipitation events caused by the cold fronts may be significant, depending on the moisture in the atmosphere during the passage. The tropical storms generally produce a significant amount of precipitation. A few inches of rainfall in 24 hours is very common along the track because the tropical storms generally carry a large amount of moisture.

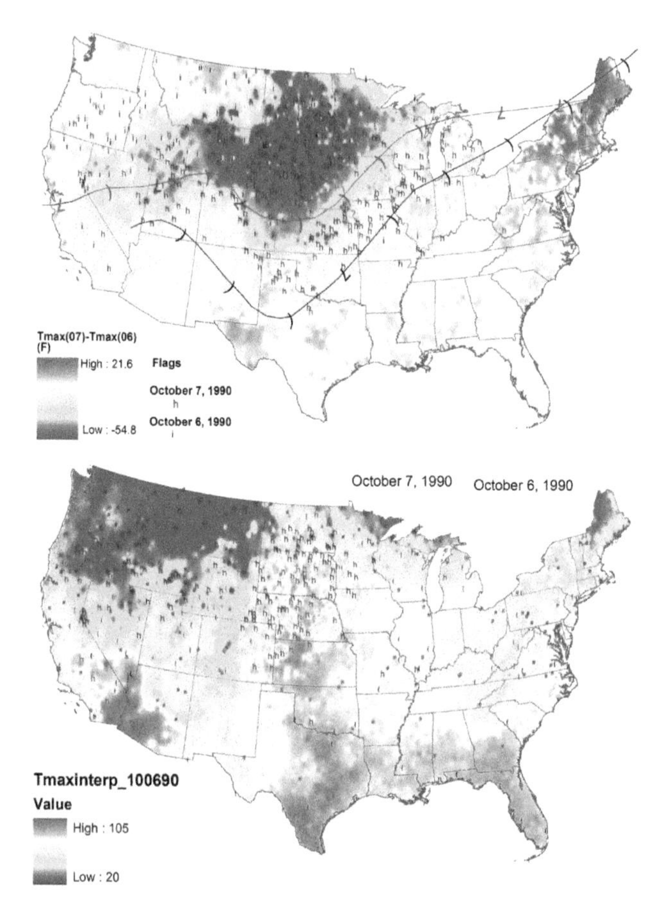

Figure 6. Spatial patterns of flagged records for cold front events and related fronts. The temperature map is the interpolated maximum temperature difference between October 6 and October 7, 1990. The color front is on October 7, and the black one is on October 6. The flags are the QA failures on that day.

5.6. Resetting the flags for cold front events and hurricanes

Some measurements during the cold front and the hurricane were valid but flagged as outliers due to the effect of QC tests during times of large temperature changes caused by the cold front [illegible] and the heavy precipitation occurring in hurricanes. A simple spatial scheme was developed to recognize regions where flags have been set due to Type I errors. The stations along the cold front may experience the mixed population where some stations have been affected by the cold fronts and others have not. A complex pattern recognition method can be applied to identify the influence zone of the cold fronts through the temperature changes (e.g. using some methods described in Jain et al, 2000). In our work, we use the simple rule to reset the flag given that significant temperature changes occur when the cold front passes. The mean and the standard deviation of the temperature change can be calculated as:

$$\overline{\Delta T} = \frac{1}{n}\sum_{i=1}^{n}\Delta T_i \tag{7}$$

$$\sigma_{\Delta T}{}^2 = \frac{1}{n}\sum_{i=0}^{n}(\Delta T_i * \Delta T_i) - \overline{\Delta T} * \overline{\Delta T} \tag{8}$$

where $\overline{\Delta T}$ is the mean temperature change of the reference stations, ΔT_i is the temperature change at the ith station for the current day, n is the number of neighboring stations, and $\sigma_{\Delta T}$ is the standard deviation of the temperature change for the current day. A second round test is applied to records that were flagged in the first round:

$$\overline{\Delta T} - f'\sigma_{\Delta T} \le \Delta T \le \overline{\Delta T} + f'\sigma_{\Delta T} \tag{9}$$

where ΔT is the difference between maximum/minimum air temperature for the current day and the last day. The cutoff value f' takes a value of 3.0. The test results with this refinement for T_{max} are shown in Fig. 7 for Oct. 7, 1990. The results obtained using the refinements described in this section were labeled "modified SRT" and the results using the original SRT were labeled "original SRT" in Fig. 7 and 8. Of the 291 flags originally noted only 41 flags remain after the reset phase. The daily temperature drops more than 20 °F at most stations where the flags were reset and the largest drop is 55 °F.

For the heavy precipitation events, we compare the amount of precipitation at neighboring stations to see whether heavy precipitation occurred. We use a similar approach as for temperature to check the number of neighboring stations that have significant precipitation,

$$\zeta = count(p_i \ge p_{threshold}) \tag{10}$$

where the p_i is the daily precipitation amount at a neighboring station, and $p_{threshold}$ is a threshold beyond which we recognize that a significant precipitation event has occurred at the neighboring station, e.g. 1 in. When $\zeta \geq 2$and$p p_{high}$, we reset the flag. Here p is the precipitation amount of the current station, and p_{high} is the upper threshold beyond which the threshold will flag the measurement. Fig.8 shows maps of flags after the reset process. Of the 78 flags originally noted only 41 flags remain after the reset phase. Most of the remaining flags are due to the precipitation being higher than the upper threshold.

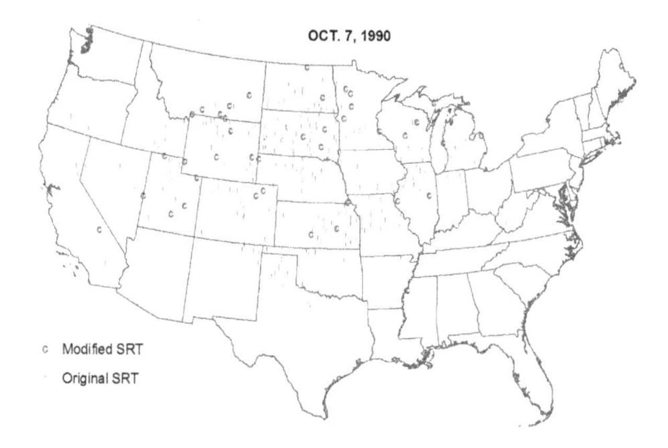

Figure 7. All points shown were flagged by the original SRT method while the red points were those that are flagged by the modified SRT method for maximum daily Temperature. Blue symbols are those that are reset by the modified SRT method.

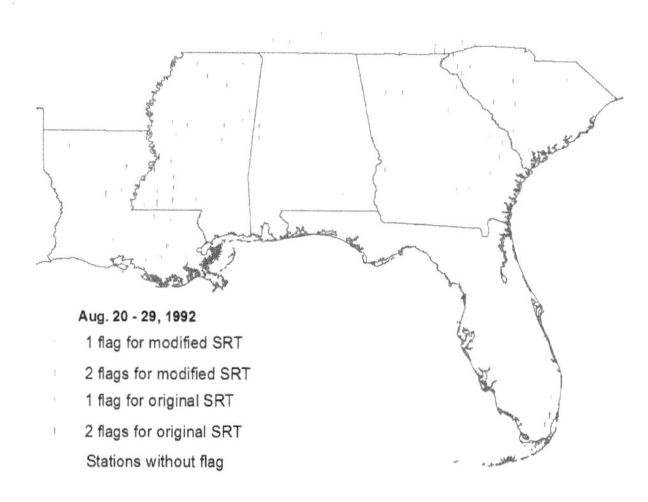

Figure 8. This is the reset of flags for the Andrew 1992 hurricane. The flags are the cumulative flags starting from Aug. 20 to Aug. 29, 1992. The flags by the modified SRT method overlay the flags by the original SRT method.

Flags for the Andrew 1992 hurricane. The flags are the cumulative flags starting from Aug. 20 to Aug. 29, 1992. The flags by the modified SRT method overlay the flags by the original SRT method.

6. Multiple interval methods based on measurements from reference stations for precipitation.

One QC approach involved developing threshold quantification methods to identify a subset of data consisting of potential outliers in the precipitation observations with the aim of reducing the manual checking workload. This QC method for precipitation was developed based on the empirical statistical distributions underlying the observations.

The search for precipitation quality control (QC) methods has proven difficult. The high spatial and temporal variability associated with precipitation data causes high uncertainty and edge creep when regression-based approaches are applied. Precipitation frequency distributions are generally skewed rather than normally distributed. The commonly assumed normal distribution in QC methods is not a good representation of the actual distribution of precipitation and is inefficient in identifying the outliers.

The SRTmethod is able to identify many of the errant data values but the rate of finding errant values to that of making type I errors is conservatively 1:6. This is not acceptable because it would take excessive manpower to check all the flagged values that are generated in a nationwide network. For example, the number of precipitation observations from the cooperative network in a typical day is 4000. Using an error rate of 2% and considering the type I error rate indicates that several hundred values may be flagged, requiring substantial personnel resources for assessment.

(29) found the use of a single gamma distribution fit to all precipitation data was ineffective. A second test, the multiple intervals gamma distribution (MIGD) method, was introduced. It assumed that meteorological conditions that produce a certain range in average precipitation at surrounding stations will produce a predictable range at the target station. The MIGD method sorts data into bins according to the average of precipitation at neighboring stations; then, for the events in a specific bin, an associated gamma distribution is derived by fit to the same events at the target station. The new gamma distributions can then be used to establish the threshold for QC according to the user-selected probability of exceedance. We also employed the *Q* test for precipitation (20) using a metric based on comparisons with neighboring stations. The performance of the three approaches was evaluated by assessing the fraction of "known" errors that can be identified in a seeded error dataset(18). The single gamma distribution and *Q*-test approach were found to be relatively efficient at identifying extreme precipitation values as potential outliers. However, the MIGD method outperforms the other two QC methods. This method identifies more seeded errors and results in fewer Type I errors than the other methods.

6.1. Estimation of parameters for distribution of precipitation and thresholds from the Gama distribution

The Gamma distribution was employed to represent the distribution of precipitation. While other functions may provide a better overall fit to precipitation data our goal is to establish a reasonable threshold on values beyond which further checking will be required to determine if the value is an outlier or simply an extreme precipitation event. The precipitation events are fit to a Gamma distribution,$G(\gamma, \beta)$. The shape and scale parameters γ, β can be estimated from the precipitation events following (21) and (13),

$$\gamma = \frac{\overline{X}^2}{s^2} \tag{11}$$

$$\beta = \frac{s^2}{\overline{X}} \tag{12}$$

where$\overline{X}$ and s are the sample mean and the sample standard deviation, respectively.

The data for each station in the Gamma distribution test include all precipitation events on a daily basis for a year. The parameters for left-censored (0 values excluded) Gamma distributions, on a monthly basis, are also calculated, based on the precipitation events for individual months in the historical record. To ascertain the representativeness of the Gamma distribution, the precipitation value for the corresponding percentiles (P): 99, 99.9, 99.99, and 99.999% were computed from the Gamma distribution and compared with the precipitation values for given percentiles based on ranking (original data).

The criterion for a threshold test approach can be written as,

$$x(j,t) < I(p) \tag{13}$$

where$x(j,t)$ is the observed daily precipitation on day t at station j and $I(p)$ is the threshold daily precipitation for a given probability, p (=P/100), calculated using the Gamma distribution. A value not meeting this criterion is noted as a potential outlier (the shaded area to the right of the p=0.995 value for the distribution for all precipitation events in Fig. 9). The test function uses the one-sided test for precipitation, a non-negative variable.

6.2. Multiple interval range limit gamma distribution test for precipitation (MIGD)

Analysis has shown that precipitation data at a station can be fit to a Gamma distribution, which can then be applied to a threshold test approach. With this method only the most extreme precipitation events will be flagged as potential outliers so errant data at other points in the distribution are not identified.

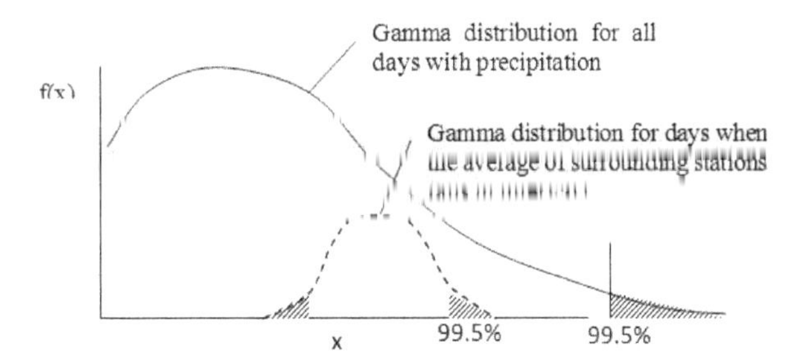

Figure 9. Schematic of gamma distribution for all daily precipitation events and for the ith interval of the MIGD approach.

The MIGD was developed to address these non-extreme points along the distribution. It assumes that meteorological conditions that produce a certain range in average precipitation at surrounding stations will produce a predictable range at the target station. Our concept is to develop a family of Gamma distributions for the station of interest and to selectively apply the distributions based on specific criteria. The average precipitation for each day is calculated for neighboring stations during a time period (e.g. 30 years). These values are ranked and placed into n bins with an equal number of values in each. The range for n intervals can be obtained from the cumulative probabilities of neighboring average time series, $\{0, 1/n, 2/n, \ldots, n\text{-}1/n, 1\}$. For the ith interval all corresponding precipitation values at the station of interest (target station) are gathered and parameters for the gamma distribution estimated. This process is repeated for each of the n intervals resulting in a family of Gamma curves (G_i). The operational QC involves the application of the threshold test where the gamma distribution for a given day is selected from the family of curves based on the average precipitation for the neighboring stations. Each interval can be defined as$(\xi(p(i/n)), \xi(p((i+1)/n))]$, where $p(i/n)$is the cumulative probability associated with i/n, i=0 to n-1, and $\xi(p(i/n))$ is the neighboring stations' average for a given cumulative probability.

Now for each precipitation event, x, at the station of interest, the neighboring stations' average is calculated. If the average precipitation falls in the interval$(\xi(p(i/n)), \xi(p((i+1)/n))]$, then G_i is used to form a test:

$$G_i(1-p) < x(j,t) < G_i(p) \tag{14}$$

where p is a probability in the range (0.5, 1), and the $G_i(p)$ is the precipitation value for the given probability p in the gamma distribution associated with the ith interval. This equation forms a two sided test. Any value that does not satisfy this test will be treated as an outlier for further manual checking. The intervals and the estimation of this method were implemented using *R* statistical software (19).

The results indicate that the Gamma distribution is well suited for deriving appropriate thresholds for a particular precipitation event. The calculated extreme values provide a good basis for identifying extreme outliers in the precipitation observations. The inclusion of all precipitation events reduces the data requirements for the quantification of extreme events which generally requires a long time series of observations (e.g. using Gumbel distribution.) Using the approach based on the Gamma distribution, a suitable representation of the distribution of precipitation can be obtained with only a few years of observation, as is the case with newly established automatic weather stations, e.g. Climate Reference Network. Further study is required for probability selection in the Gamma distribution approach.

sname	range	lower	upper	q999	q995	q99	q975	q95	q9	q1	q05	q025	q01	q005
028820	0~0.0510	0	0.0510	0.8441	0.6332	0.5431	0.4251	0.3369	0.2502	0.0055	0.0021	0.0008	0.0002	9.39E-05
028820	0.0510~0.1111	0.0510	0.1111	1.1533	0.8704	0.7493	0.5903	0.4711	0.3532	0.0097	0.0040	0.0017	0.0005	0.0002
028820	0.1111~0.1899	0.1111	0.1899	1.2989	0.9896	0.8567	0.6816	0.5495	0.4181	0.0156	0.0071	0.0033	0.0012	0.0006
028820	0.1899~0.3326	0.1899	0.3326	1.8631	1.4162	1.2243	0.9717	0.7815	0.5925	0.0206	0.0092	0.0042	0.0015	0.0007
028820	0.3326~2.1216	0.3326	2.1216	2.8514	2.1861	1.8996	1.5210	1.2346	0.9484	0.0429	0.0208	0.0102	0.0040	0.0020

Table 5. Multiple gamma distributions (n=5) for the Multiple Interval Gamma Distribution (MIGD) method at Tucson, AZ. Lower and upper represent the upper and lower limits of each bin for surrounding station averages. The precipitation threshold for the target station can be selected from q999, q995, q99, q975, q95, q9, q1,q05,q025,q01, q005, and q001 as these are associated with gamma distribution for the station of interest.

A simple gamma distribution can be fit to the daily precipitation values at a station. Upper thresholds can be set based on the cumulative probability of the precipitation distribution. This single gamma distribution (SGD) test will address the most extreme values of precipitation and flag them for further testing. However, to address non-extreme values of precipitation that are not out on the tail of the SGD another approach is needed. We have formulated the multiple interval gamma distribution test (MIGD) for this purpose. The main assumption is that the meteorological conditions that produce a certain range in average precipitation at surrounding stations will produce a predictable range of precipitation at the target station. It does not estimate the precipitation at the target station but estimates the range into which the precipitation should fit.

The average precipitation for each day is calculated for neighboring stations during a historical period, say 30 years. These values are then ranked and placed into n bins with an equal number of values in each. For all the values in a given bin, the daily precipitation at the target station are gathered and a gamma distribution formed. The process is repeated n times once for each bin resulting in a family of gamma distribution curves. A separate family of curves can be derived for each month or each season. In operation, the daily average of the precipitation at surrounding stations is calculated and used to point to the n'th gamma distribution which in turn provides thresholds against which to test for that day. For instance, the upper threshold can be selected to correspond with the cumulative probability for the n'th gamma distribution. The user is able to specify the threshold according the cumulative probability. For example we can be 99.5 % confident that values will not exceed the corresponding value on the cumulative probability curve. Values that exceed this are not necessarily wrong but flagged for further review. The MIGD will find more precipitation values that need to be reviewed than the single gamma distribution test.

Table 5 provides an example of the MIGD for n=5 at Tucson, AZ, USA. We update this type of information on an annual basis. If the precipitation value falls outside the q value of a selected confidence level, we mark the value as an outlier. For example, Suppose we select q999 for our confidence. The precipitation on August 2, 1987 was 1.3 inches while the average of neighboring stations had a value of 0.06 inches. The average falls between lower and upper in the 2nd row, n=2, ie.0.05, 0.11. The rainfall value (1.3 inches) is larger than the q999 threshold (1.15 inches) thus we can say we are 99.9 % confident that the rainfall is an outlier and it should be flagged for further manual examination. Note that 1.3 inches is in no way an extreme precipitation value but, it's validity can be challenged on the basis of the MIGD test.

One other QC method for precipitation test is the Q-test (20). The Q-test approach serves as a tool to discriminate between extreme precipitation and outliers and it has proven to minimize the manual examination of precipitation by choice of parameters that identify the most likely outliers (20). The performance of both the Gamma distribution test and the Q-test is relatively weak with respect to identifying the seeded errors. The Q-Test is different from the Gamma distribution method because the Q-Test uses both the historical data and measurements from neighboring stations while the simple implementation of the Gamma distribution method only uses the data from the station of interest.

The MIGD method is a more complex implementation of the Gamma distribution that uses historical data and measurements from neighboring stations to partition a station's precipitation values into separate populations. The MIGD method shows promise and outperforms other QC methods for precipitation. This method identifies more seeded errors and creates fewer Type I errors than the other methods. MIGD will be used as an operational tool in identifying the outliers for precipitation in ACIS. However, the fraction of errors identified by the MIGD method varies for different probabilities and among the different stations. Network operators, data managers, and scientist who plan to use MIGD to identify potential precipitation outliers can perform a similar analysis (sort the data into bins and derive the gamma distribution coefficients for each interval) over their geographic region to choose an optimum probability level.

7. Quality control of the NCDC dataset to create a serially complete dataset.

Development of continuous and high-quality climate datasets is essential to populate Web-distributed databases (17) and to serve as input to Decision Support Systems (e.g., 27).

Serially complete data are necessary as input to many risk assessments related to human endeavor including the frequency analysis associated with heavy rains, severe heat, severe cold, and drought. Continuous data are also needed to understand the climate impacts on crop yield, and ecosystem production. The National Drought Mitigation Center (NDMC) and the High Plains Regional Climate Center (HPRCC) at the University of Nebraska are developing a new drought atlas. The last drought atlas (1994) was produced with the data from 1119 stations ending in 1992. The forthcoming drought atlas will include additional stations and will update the analyses, maps, and figures through the period 1994 to the present time. A list was compiled from the Applied Climate Information System (ACIS) for stations with a length of at least 40 years of observations for all three variables: precipitation (PRCP), maximum (Tmax), and minimum (Tmin) temperatures. Paper records were scrutinized to identify reported, but previously non-digitized data to reduce, to the extent possible, the number of missing data. A list of 2144 stations was compiled for the sites that met the criterion of at least 40 years data with less than two months continuous missing gaps for at least one of the three variables. The remaining missing data in the dataset were supplemented by the estimates obtained from the measurements made at nearby stations. The spatial regression test (SRT) and the inverse distance weighted (IDW) method were adopted in a dynamic data filling procedure to provide these estimates. The replacement of missing values follows a reproducible process that uses robust estimation procedures and results in a serially complete data set (SCD) for 2144 stations that provide a firm basis for climate analysis. Scientists who have used more qualitative or less sophisticated quantitative QC techniques may wish to use this data set so that direct comparisons to other studies that used this SCD can be made without worry about how differences in missing dataprocedures would influence the results. A drought atlas based on data from the SCD will provide decision makers more support in their risk management needs.

After identifying stations with a long-term (at least 40 years) continuous (no data gaps longer than two months) dataset of Tmax, Tmin, and/or PRCP for a total of 2144 stations, the missing values in the original dataset retrieved from ACIS were filled to the extent possible with the keyed data from paper record and the estimates using the SRT and IDW methods. Two implementations of SRT were applied in this study. The short-window (60 days) implementation provides the best estimates based on the most recent information available for constructing the regression. The second implementation of SRT fills the long gaps, e.g. gaps longer than one month using the data available on a yearly basis. The IDW method was adopted to fill any remaining missing data after the two implementations of SRT.

This is the first serially complete data set where a statement of confidence can be associated with many of the estimates, ie. SRT estimates. The RMSE is less than 1F in most cases and thus we are 95% confident that the value, if available, would lie between ±2F of the estimate. This data set is available [1] to interested parties and can be used in crop models, assessment of severe heat, cold, and dryness. Probabilities related to extreme rainfall for flooding and erosion potential can be derived along with indices to reflect impact on livestock production. The data set is offered as an option to distributing raw data to the users who need this level of spatial and temporal coverage but are not well positioned to spend time and resources to fill gaps with acceptable estimates.

Analysis based on the long-term dataset will best reveal the regional and large scale climatic variability in the continental U.S., making this an ideal data set for the development of a new drought atlas and associated drought index calculations. Future data observations can be easily appended to this SCD with the dynamic data filling procedures described herein.

---

1 Contact the High Plains Regional Climate Center at 402-472-6709

8. Issues relating QC to gridded datasets,

Gridded datasets are sometimes used in QC but, we caution against this for the following reasons.New datasets created from inverse distance weighted methods or krigging suffer from uncertainties. The values at a grid point are usually not "true"measurements but are interpolated values from the measurements at nearby stations in the weather network. Thus, the values at the grid points are susceptible to bias. When further interpolation is made to a given location within the grid, bias will again exist at the specific location between the gridded values..Fig.10provides an example of potential bias. Outside of a gridded data set the target location would give a large weight to the value at station 5. However, if the radius used for the gridded data is as in the Fig.10, then the closest station to the target station (5) will not be included in the grid-based estimation.

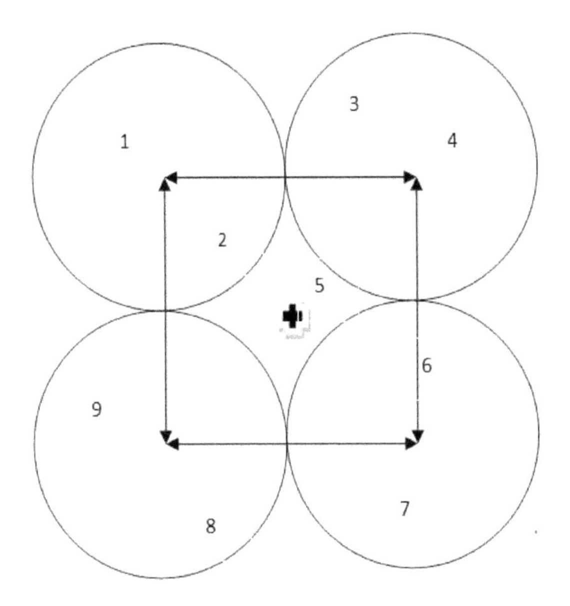

Figure 10. An example of station distribution used in the grid method.

9. Quality control of high temporal resolution datasets

The Oklahoma Mesonet (http://www.mesonet.org/) measures and archives weather conditions at 5-minute intervals (Shafer et al., 2000). The quality control system used in the network starts from the raw data of the measurements for the high temporal resolution data. A set of QC tools was developed to routinely maintain data of the Mesonet. These tools depend on the status of hardware and measurement flag sets built in the climate data system.The Climate Reference Network (CRN, Baker et al. 2004) is another example of the QC of high frequency data, which installs multiple sensors for each variable to guarantee the continuous operation of the weather station and thus the quality control can also rely on the multiple measurements of a single variable. This method is efficient to detect the instrumental failures or other disturbances; however the cost of such a network may be prohibitive for non-research or operational networks. The authors of this chapter also carried out QC on a high temporal resolution dataset in the Beaufort and Chukchi Sea regions. Surface meteorological data from more than 200 stations in a variety of observing networks and various stand-alone projects were obtained for the MMS Beaufort and Chukchi Seas Modeling Study (Phase II). Many stations have a relatively short period of record (i.e. less than 10 years).The traditional basic QC procedures were developed and tested for a daily data and found in need of improvement for the high temporal resolution data. In the modification, the time series of the maximum and the minimum were calculated from the high resolution data. The mean and standard deviation of the maximum and the minimum can then be calculated from the time series (e.g max and min temperatures) as the (u_x, s_x) and (u_n, s_n), respectively. The equation (6) using ($u_x + f\ s_x$) and ($u_n - f\ s_n$) forms limits defined by the upper limits of the maximum and lower limits of the minimum. The value falling outside the limits will be flagged as an outlier for further manual checking. Similarly, the diurnal change of a variable (e.g. temperature) was calculated from the high resolution (hourly or sub-hourly) data. The mean and standard deviation calculated from the diurnal changes will form the limits.

The traditional quality control methods were improved for examining the high temporal resolution data, to avoid intensive manual reviewing which is not timely or cost efficient. The identified problems in the dataset demonstrate that the improved methods did find considerable errors in the raw data including the time errors (e.g. month being great than 12). These newtools offer a dataset that, after manual checking of the flagged data, can be givin a statement of confidence. The level of confidence can be selected by the user, prior to QC.

The applied in-station limit tests can successfully identify outliers in the dataset. However, spatial tests based information from the neighboring stations is more robust in many cases and identifies errors or outliers in the dataset when strong correlation exists. The good relationship between the measurements at station pairs demonstrates that there is a potential opportunity to successfully apply the spatial regression test (SRT, 18) to the stations which measure the same variables (i.e. air temperature orwind speed). The short term measurements at some stations may not be efficiently QC'ed with only the three methods described in this work. One example is the dew point measurements at the first-order station Iultin-in-Chukot. More than 90 percent of the dew point measurements were flagged, because the parameters for QC'ing the variable used the state wide parameters which cannot reflect the microclimate of each station.

10. Summary and Conclusions

Quality control (QC) methods can never provide total proof that a data point is good or bad. Type I errors (false positives) or Type II errors (false negatives) can occur and result in labeling of good data as bad and bad data as good respectively. Decreasing the number of Type I and Type II errors is difficult because often a push to decrease Type I errors will result in an unintended increase inType II errors and vice versa. We have derived a spatial technique to introduce thresholds associated with user selected probabilities (i.e. select 99.7% as the level of confidence that a data value is an outlier before labeling it as bad and/or replacing it with an estimate.) We base this technique on statistical regression in the neighborhood of the data in question and call it the Spatial Regression Test (SRT). Observations taken in a network are often affected by the same factors. In weather applications individual stations in a network are generally exposed to air masses in much the same way as are neighboring stations. Thus, temperatures in the vicinity move up and down together and the correlation between data in the same neighborhood is very high.Similarly seasonal forcings on this neighborhood (e.g. the day to day and seasonal solar irradiance) are essentially the same. We have defined a neighborhood for a station as those nearby stations that are best correlated to it. We found that the SRT method is an improvement over conventional inverse distance weighting estimates (IDW). A huge benefit of the SRT method is it's ability to remove systematic biases in the data estimation process. Additionally, the method allows a user selected threshold on the probability as contrasted to the IDW. Although the SRT estimates are similar to IDW estimates over smooth terrain, SRT estimates are notably superior over complex terrain (mountains) and in the vicinity of other climate forcing (e.g. ocean/land boundaries). Gridded data sets that result from IDW, Kriging or most other interpolation schemes do not provide unbiased estimates. Even when grid spacing is decreased to a point where the complexity of the land surface is well represented there remains two problems: what is the microclimate of the nearest observation points and what is the transfer function between points. This is a future challenge for increasing the quality of data sets and the estimation of data between observation sites.

Author details

Kenneth Hubbard*, Jinsheng You and Martha Shulski

*Address all correspondence to: khubbard1@unl.edu

High Plains Regional Climate Center, University of Nebraska, Lincoln, NE, USA

References

[1] Barnett, V., & Lewis, T. (1994). *Outliers in Statistical Data* (3 ed.), J. Wiley and Sons, 604.

[2] Camargo, M. B. P., & Hubbard, K. G. (1999). Spatial and temporal variability of daily weather variables in sub-humid and semi-arid areas of the U.S. *High Plains.Ag.and Forest Meteor.*, 93, 141-148.

[3] Eischeid, J. K., Baker, C. B., Karl, T., & Diaz, H. F. (1995). The quality control of long-term climatological data using objective data analysis. *J. Appl. Meteor.*, 34, 2787-2795.

[4] Gandin, L. S. (1988). Complex quality control of meteorological observations. *Mon. Wea. Rev.*, 116, 1137-1156.

[5] Guttman, N., Karl, C., Reek, T., & Shuler, V. (1988). Measuring the performance of data validators. *Bull. Amer. Meteor. Soc.*, 69(12), 1448-1452.

[6] Guttman, N., & Quayler, R. G. (1990). A review of Cooperative temperature data validation. *J. Atmos. Ocean. Tech.*, 7(2), 334-339.

[7] Hubbard, K. G., & You, J. (2005). Sensitivity analysis of quality assurance using spatial regression approach-a case study of maximum/minimum air temperature. *J. Atmos. And Oceanic Technology.*, 22(10), 1520-1530.

[8] Hubbard, K. G., Goddard, S., Sorensen, W. D., Wells, N., & Osugi, T. T. (2005). Performance of quality assurance procedures for an Applied Climate Information System. *J. Atmos. Ocean. Tech.*, 22(1), 105-112.

[9] Meek, D. W., & Hatfield, J. L. (1994). Data quality checking for single station meteorological databases. *Agric. For. Meteor.*, 69, 85-109.

[10] Shafer, M. A., Fiebrich, C. A., Arndt, D., Fredrickson, S. E., & Hughes, T. W. (2000). Quality assurance procedures in the Oklahoma Mesonetwork. *J. Atmos. Ocean. Tech.*, 17, 474-494.

[11] Wade, C. G. (1987). A quality control program for surface mesometeorological data. *J. Atmos. Ocean. Tech.*, 4, 435-453.

[12] Eischeid, J. K., Baker, C. B., Karl, T., & Diaz, H. F. (1995). The quality control of long-term climatological data using objective data analysis. *J. Appl. Meteor.*, 34, 2787-2795.

[13] Evans, M. , Hastings, N., & Peacock, B. (2000). *Statistical Distributions* (3rd. Ed.), John Wiley and Sons, 221.

[14] Gandin, L. S. (1988). Complex quality control of meteorological observations. *Mon. Wea. Rev.*, 116, 1137-1156.

[15] Guttman, N. V., & Quayle, R. G. (1990). A review of cooperative temperature data validation. *J. Atmos. and Oceanic Tech.*, 7, 334-339.

[16] Hubbard, K. G. (2001). Multiple station quality control procedures. *In Automated Weather Stations for Applications in Agriculture and Water Resources Management. AGM-3 WMO./TD* [1074], 248.

[17] Hubbard, K. G., De Gaetano, A. T., & Robbins, K. D. (2004). Announcing a Modern Applied Climatic Information System (ACIS). *Bull. Amer. Meteorol. Soc.*, 85(6), 811-812.

[18] Hubbard, K. G., Goddard, S., Sorensen, W. D., Wells, N., & Osugi, T. T. (2005). Performance of Quality Assurance Procedures for an Applied Climate Information System. *J. Atmos. and Oceanic Tech.*, 22, 105-112.

[19] Ihaka, R., & Gentleman, R. (1996). R: A language for data analysis and graphics. *J. of Computational and Graphical Statistics*, 5, 299-314.

[20] Kunkel, K. E., Easterling, D. R., Hubbard, K., Redmond, K, Andsager, K, Kruk, M. C., & Spinar, M. L. (2005). Quality control of pre-1948 cooperative network observer data. *J. Atmos. Oceanic Technol*, 22, 1691-1705.

[21] Johnson, N. L., Kotz, S., & Balakrishnan, N. (1994). *Continuous Univariate Distributions Volumes I and II* (2nd. Ed.), John Wiley and Sons, 761.

[22] Martinez, J. E., Fiebrich, C. A., & Shafer, M. A. (2004). The Value of a Quality Assurance Meteorologist. Seattle, WA. *14th Conference on Applied Climatology, The 84th AMS Annual Meeting*.

[23] Meek, D. W., & Hatfield, J. L. (1994). Data quality checking for single station meteorological databases. *Agric. and Forest Meteor.*, 69, 85-109.

[24] National Weather Service. (1987). *Cooperative Program Management, Weather Service Operations Manual B-17 (revised)*, Silver Spring, MD, National Oceanic and Atmospheric Administration, 50.

[25] Reek, T., Doty, S. R., & Owen, T. W. (1992). A Deterministic Approach to the Validation of Historical Daily Temperature and Precipitation Data from the Cooperative Network. *Bull. Amer. Meteorolog. Soc.*, 73(6), 753-765.

[26] Wade, C. G. (1987). A quality control program for surface mesometeorological data. *J. Atmos. and Oceanic Tech.*, 4, 435-453.

[27] Westphal, K. S., Vogel, R. M., Kirshen, P., & Chapra, S. C. (2003). Decision Support System for Adaptive Water Supply Management. *Journal of Water Resources Planning and Management*, 129(3), 165-177.

[28] You, J., & Hubbard, K. G. (2006). Quality Control of Weather Data during Extreme Events. *J. Atmos. and Oceanic Tech.*, 23(2), 184-197.

[29] You, J. K., Hubbard, G., & Goddard, S. (2007). Comaparison of methods for spatially estimating station temperatures in a quality control system. *International J. of Climatology*, 28, 777-787, DOI: joc.1571.

Chapter 2

New Models of Acceptance Sampling Plans

Mohammad Saber Fallah Nezhad

Additional information is available at the end of the chapter

1. Introduction

Acceptance sampling is a procedure used for sentencing incoming batches. Sampling plan consist of a sample size and a decision making rule. The sample size is the number of items to sample or the number of measurements to take. The decision making rule involves the acceptance threshold and a description of how to use the sample result to accept or reject the lot. Acceptance sampling plans are also practical tools for quality control applications, which involve quality contracting on product orders between the vendor and the buyer. Those sampling plans provide the vendor and the buyer rules for lot sentencing while meeting their preset requirements on product quality. Scientific sampling plans are the primary tools for quality and performance management in industry today. In an industrial plant, sampling plans are used to decide either to accept or reject a received batch of items. With attribute sampling plans, these accept/reject decisions are based on a count of the number of defective items. The sample size is assumed constant in traditional sampling plans.

In this section, several new decision making policies for the acceptance sampling problem are introduced. The objective of these models is to find constant control thresholds for lot sentencing problem.

The single stage acceptance sampling plan based on the control threshold policy is presented in section 2, the acceptance sampling policy based on number of successive conforming items is presented in section 3, and acceptance sampling policy using the minimum angle method is presented in sections 4. Acceptance sampling policy based on cumulative sum of conforming Items run lengths comes in section 5 and acceptance sampling policy based on Bayesian inference comes in section 6. Finally the chapter is concluded in section 7.

2. Single Stage Acceptance Sampling Plan based on the Control Threshold Policy [1]

We suppose a batch of size n is received which its proportion of the detectives items is equal to p. For a batch of size n, random variable Y is defined as the number of inspected items and z is defined as the number of items classified as 'defective' after inspection. The number of inspected items has an upper threshold equal to m. For $Y = 1, 2, \ldots, m$ inspected items ($m \le n$) the batch will be rejected if $x \le z$ where x is the upper control level for batch acceptance. In the other words, when the number of defective items in the inspected items gets more than the control threshold x then decision making process stops and the batch is rejected.

The probability distribution function of Y is determined by the following equations,

$$\Pr\{Y\} = \begin{cases} \begin{cases} \sum_{z=0}^{x} \Pr\{z\} = \\ \Pr\{z \le x-1\} + \Pr\{z = x\} \\ = \sum_{z=0}^{x-1} \binom{m}{z} p^z (1-p)^{m-z} + \\ \binom{m-1}{x-1} p^x (1-p)^{m-x} \end{cases} & Y = m \\ \binom{Y-1}{x-1} p^x (1-p)^{Y-x} & x \le Y < m \end{cases} \tag{1}$$

In Eq. (1), $Y = m$ indicates that all items are inspected therefore, the number of defective items has been less than x or x_{th} defective item has been m_{th} inspected item. For the case $x \le Y m$, x_{th} defective item has been Y_{th} inspected item thus, the probability distribution function of Y follows a negative binomial distribution. The expected mean of the number of inspected items is determined as follows:

$$\begin{aligned} E[Y]_x &= m\sum_{z=0}^{x-1} \binom{m}{z} p^z(1-p)^{m-z} + m\binom{m-1}{x-1} p^x(1-p)^{m-x} \\ &+ \sum_{Y=x}^{m-1} Y\binom{Y-1}{x-1} p^x(1-p)^{Y-x} = m\sum_{z=0}^{x-1}\binom{m}{z} p^z(1-p)^{m-z} + \\ &\sum_{Y=x}^{m} Y\binom{Y-1}{x-1} p^x(1-p)^{Y-x} \end{aligned} \tag{2}$$

Since $\Pr\{Y\} = \binom{Y-1}{x-1} p^x(1-p)^{Y-x} \quad x \le Y m$ is a negative binomial distribution thus using the approximation method of estimating negative binomial probabilities with Poisson distribution [2], following is concluded,

$$\Pr\{Y\} = Poisson(\lambda) = \frac{e^{-\lambda}\lambda^{Y-x}}{\Gamma(Y-x+1)} \tag{3}$$

where $\lambda = x\frac{1-p}{p}$ is the parameter of Poisson distribution. In order to improve the accuracy of this approximation, m and x should be sufficiently large numbers. Using the above approximation method, following is concluded,

$$E[Y]_x \simeq m\sum_{z=0}^{x-1}\binom{m}{z}p^z(1-p)^{m-z} + \sum_{Y=x}^{m} Y\frac{e^{-\lambda}\lambda^{Y-x}}{\Gamma(Y-x+1)} \tag{4}$$

Now, let P_x denotes the probability of rejecting the batch. The batch is rejected if the number of defective items is more than or equal to x thus the value of P_x is determined by the following equation,

$$P_x = \sum_{z=x}^{m}\binom{m}{z}p^z(1-p)^{m-z} \tag{5}$$

In order to calculate the total cost, including the cost of rejecting the batch, the cost of inspection and the cost of defective items, assume R is the cost of rejecting the batch, c is the inspection cost of one item and c' is the cost of one defective item, so the total cost, C_x, is determined by conditioning C_x on two events of rejecting or accepting the batch, thus the objective function is written as follows:

$$\begin{aligned}&C_x = E\left(C_x \middle| \text{Reject the batch}\right)P\left(\text{Reject the batch}\right) + \\ &E\left(C_x \middle| \text{Accept the batch}\right)P\left(\text{Accept the batch}\right) = P_x\left(R + cE[Y]_x\right) + \\ &\left(npc' + cE[Y]_x\right)\left(1-P_x\right) = P_xR + npc'\left(1-P_x\right) + cE[Y]_x\end{aligned} \tag{6}$$

Thus we have,

$$\begin{aligned}&C_x = P_xR + npc'(1-P_x) + mc\sum_{z=0}^{x-1}\binom{m}{z}p^z(1-p)^{m-z} \\ &+c\sum_{Y=x}^{m} Y\frac{e^{-\lambda}\lambda^{Y-x}}{\Gamma(Y-x+1)} = R\sum_{z=x}^{m}\binom{m}{z}p^z(1-p)^{m-z} \\ &+\sum_{z=0}^{x-1}\binom{m}{z}p^z(1-p)^{m-z}(npc' + mc) + c\sum_{Y=x}^{m} Y\frac{e^{-\lambda}\lambda^{Y-x}}{\Gamma(Y-x+1)}\end{aligned} \tag{7}$$

In Eq. (7), $cE[Y]_x$ is the total cost of inspection and npc' is the total cost of defective items. The optimal value of x is determined by minimizing the value of objective function C_x. Using the optimization methods, it is concluded that.

$$\Delta C_x = C_x - C_{x-1} = R\sum_{z=x}^{m}\binom{m}{z}p^z(1-p)^{m-z} + (mc+npc')\sum_{z=0}^{x-1}\binom{m}{z}p^z(1-p)^{m-z} + c\sum_{Y=x}^{m}Y\frac{e^{-\lambda}\lambda^{Y-x}}{\Gamma(Y-x+1)} = -\left(\begin{array}{l} R\sum_{z=x-1}^{m}\binom{m}{z}p^z(1-p)^{m-z} + \\ (mc+npc')\sum_{z=0}^{x-2}\binom{m}{z}p^z(1-p)^{m-z} + \\ c\sum_{Y=x-1}^{m}Y\frac{e^{-\lambda}\lambda^{Y-x}}{\Gamma(Y-(x-1)+1)} + \end{array}\right) \tag{8}$$

To evaluate above equation, following equality is considered,

$$\sum_{Y=x}^{m}Y\frac{e^{-\lambda}\lambda^{Y-x}}{\Gamma(Y-x+1)} - \sum_{Y=x-1}^{m}Y\frac{e^{-\lambda}\lambda^{Y-(x-1)}}{\Gamma(Y-(x-1)+1)} = \sum_{Y=x}^{m}\frac{e^{-\lambda}\lambda^{Y-x}}{\Gamma(Y-x+1)} - m\frac{e^{-\lambda}\lambda^{m-(x-1)}}{\Gamma(m-(x-1)+1)} \tag{9}$$

Since m is a sufficiently large number thus the value of $m\frac{e^{-\lambda}\lambda^{m-(x-1)}}{\Gamma(m-(x-1)+1)}$ is approximately equal to zero therefore it is concluded that,

$$\Delta C_x = -R\binom{m}{x-1}p^{x-1}(1-p)^{m-(x-1)} + (mc+npc')\binom{m}{x-1}p^{x-1}(1-p)^{m-(x-1)} + c\sum_{Y=x}^{m}\frac{e^{-\lambda}\lambda^{Y-x}}{\Gamma(Y-x+1)} = (mc+npc'-R)\binom{m}{x-1}p^{x-1}(1-p)^{m-(x-1)} + c\sum_{Y=x}^{m}\frac{e^{-\lambda}\lambda^{Y-x}}{\Gamma(Y-x+1)} \tag{10}$$

To ensure that x minimizes the objective function (7), it is necessary to find the value of x that satisfies following inequalities:

$$\Delta C_{x+1} = C_{x+1} - C_x > 0,\ \Delta C_x = C_x - C_{x-1} < 0 \tag{11}$$

Hence,

$$\Delta C_{x+1} = (mc + npc' - R)\binom{m}{x} p^{x}(1-p)^{m-x} + c\sum_{Y=x+1}^{m} \frac{e^{-\lambda}\lambda^{Y-(x+1)}}{\Gamma(Y-(x+1)+1)} > 0$$
$$\Delta C_{x} = (mc + npc' - R)\binom{m}{x-1} p^{x-1}(1-p)^{m-(x-1)} + c\sum_{Y=x}^{m} \frac{e^{-\lambda}\lambda^{Y-x}}{\Gamma(Y-x+1)} < 0 \quad (12)$$

Now If $mc + npc' < R$, then,

$$\binom{m}{x-1} p^{x-1}(1-p)^{m-(x-1)} > \frac{c\sum_{Y=x}^{m} \frac{e^{-\lambda}\lambda^{Y-x}}{\Gamma(Y-x+1)}}{(R-(mc+npc'))} >$$
$$\frac{c\sum_{Y=x+1}^{m} \frac{e^{-\lambda}\lambda^{Y-x}}{\Gamma(Y-x+1)}}{(R-(mc+npc'))} > \binom{m}{x} p^{x}(1-p)^{m-x} \quad (13)$$

Since with increasing the value of x the value of binomial distribution with parameters m and p decreases thus according to the properties of binomial distribution, it is concluded that $x > (m+1)p$ therefore, the optimal value of $x$is determined using the following formula,

$$x = Min\left\{ \begin{array}{l} x; x > (m+1)p; \binom{m}{x-1} p^{x-1}(1-p)^{m-(x-1)} > \frac{c\sum_{Y=x}^{m} \frac{e^{-\lambda}\lambda^{Y-x}}{\Gamma(Y-x+1)}}{(R-(mc+npc'))} > \\ \frac{c\sum_{Y=x+1}^{m} \frac{e^{-\lambda}\lambda^{Y-x}}{\Gamma(Y-x+1)}}{(R-(mc+npc'))} > \binom{m}{x} p^{x}(1-p)^{m-x} \end{array} \right\} \quad (14)$$

Also The objective function, C_x, should be minimized regarding two constraints on Type-I and Type-II errors associated with the acceptance sampling plans. Type-I error is the probability of rejecting the batch when the nonconformity proportion of the batch is acceptable. Type-II error is the probability of accepting the batch when the nonconforming proportion of the batch is not acceptable. Then, in one hand, if$p=\delta_1$, the probability of rejecting the batch should be less thanα. On the other hand, in case where$p=\delta_2$, the probability of accepting the batch should be less thanβ where δ_1 is the AQL (Accepted Quality Level) and $\delta_2$is the LQL (Limiting Quality Level) andα is the probability of Type-I error and β is the probability of Type-II error in making a decision, therefore, the optimal value of $x$is determined using the following formula,

$$x = \text{Argmin}\left\{\begin{array}{l} x; x > (m+1)p; \\ \binom{m}{x-1} p^{x-1}(1-p)^{m-(x-1)} > \dfrac{c\sum_{Y=x}^{m} \frac{e^{-\lambda}\lambda^{Y-x}}{\Gamma(Y-x+1)}}{\left(R-(mc+npc')\right)}; \\ \dfrac{c\sum_{Y=x+1}^{m} \frac{e^{-\lambda}\lambda^{Y-x}}{\Gamma(Y-x+1)}}{\left(R-(mc+npc')\right)} > \binom{m}{x} p^{x}(1-p)^{m-x} \\ \sum_{z=x}^{m}\binom{m}{z}\delta_1^{z}(1-\delta_1)^{m-z} \le \alpha, \sum_{z=0}^{x-1}\binom{m}{z}\delta_2^{z}(1-\delta_2)^{m-z} \le \beta \end{array}\right\} \quad (15)$$

When $mc + npc' > R$, It is concluded that Eq. (16) is positive for all values of x so $x = 0$. In this case, if one defective item is found in an inspected sample then the batch would be rejected. In this case, the rejection cost R is less than the total cost of inspecting m items and the cost of defective items, hence rejecting the batch would be the optimal decision. However, in practice the rejection cost R is usually big enough so that, we overlooked that case.

$$\Delta C_x = (mc + npc' - R)\binom{m}{x-1} p^{x-1}(1-p)^{m-(x-1)} + c\sum_{Y=x}^{m} \frac{e^{-\lambda}\lambda^{Y-x}}{\Gamma(Y-x+1)} \quad (16)$$

3. Acceptance Sampling Policy Based on Number of Successive Conforming Items [3]

In a typical acceptance-sampling plan, when the number of conforming items between successive nonconforming items is more than an upper control threshold, the batch is accepted, and when it is less than a lower control threshold, the batch is rejected otherwise, the inspection process continues. This initiates the idea of employing a Markovian approach to model the acceptance-sampling problem. As a result, in this method, a new acceptance-sampling policy using Markovian models is proposed, in which determining the control thresholds are aimed. The notations required to model the problem at hand are given as:

N: The number of items in the batch

p: The proportion of nonconforming items in the batch

I: The cost of inspecting one item

c: The cost of one nonconforming item

R: The cost of rejecting the batch

$E(TC)$: The expected total cost of the system

$E(AC)$: The expected total cost of accepting the batch

$E(RP)$: The expected total cost of rejecting the batch

$E(I)$: The expected total cost of inspecting the items of the batch

U: The upper control threshold

L : The lower control threshold

Consider an incoming batch of N items with a proportion of nonconformities p, of which items are randomly selected for inspection and based on the number of conforming items between two successive nonconforming items, the batch is accepted, rejected, or the inspection continues. The expected total cost associated with this inspection policy can be expressed using Eq. (17).

$$E(TC)=E(AC)+E(RP)+E(I) \tag{17}$$

Let Y_i be the number of conforming items between the successive $(i-1)^{th}$ and i^{th} nonconforming items, U the upper and L the lower control thresholds. Then, if $Y_i \geq U$ the batch is accepted, if $Y_i \leq L$ the batch is rejected. Otherwise, if $L < Y_i < U$ the process of inspecting items continues. The states involved in this process can be defined as follows.

State 1: Y_i falls within two control thresholds L, i.e., $L < Y_i < U$, thus the inspection process continues.

State 2: Y_i is more than or equal the upper control threshold, i.e., $Y_i \geq U$, hence the batch is accepted.

State 3: Y_i is less than or equal the lower control threshold, i.e., $Y_i \leq L$, hence the batch is rejected.

The transition probabilities among the states can be obtained as follows.

Probability of inspecting more items $=p_{11}=\Pr\{L < Y_i < U\}$

Probability of accepting the batch $=p_{12}=\Pr\{Y_i \geq U\}$

Probability of rejecting the batch $=p_{13}=\Pr\{Y_i \leq L\}$

where the probabilities can be obtained based on the fact that the number of conforming items between the successive $(i-1)^{th}$ and i^{th} nonconforming items, Y_i, follows a geometric distribution with parameter p, i.e., $\Pr(Y_i=r)=(1-p)^r p; r=0, 1, 2, \ldots$ Then, the transition probability matrix is expressed as follows:

$$\mathbf{P} = \begin{matrix} & 1 & 2 & 3 \\ 1 & p_{11} & p_{12} & p_{13} \\ 2 & 0 & 1 & 0 \\ 3 & 0 & 0 & 1 \end{matrix} \tag{18}$$

As it can be seen, the matrix P is an absorbing Markov chain with states 2 and 3 being absorbing and state 1 being transient.

To analyze the above absorbing Markov chain, the transition probability matrix should be rearranged in the following form:

$$\begin{bmatrix} A & O \\ R & Q \end{bmatrix} \tag{19}$$

Rearranging the P matrix yields the following matrix:

$$\begin{matrix} & 2 & 3 & 1 \\ 2 & 1 & 0 & 0 \\ 3 & 0 & 1 & 0 \\ 1 & p_{12} & p_{13} & p_{11} \end{matrix} \tag{20}$$

Then, the fundamental matrix M can be obtained as follows [4],

$$M = m_{11} = (I - Q)^{-1} = \frac{1}{1 - p_{11}} = \frac{1}{1 - \Pr\{L < Y_i < U\}} \tag{21}$$

Where I is the identity matrix and m_{11} denotes the expected long-run number of times the transient state 1 is occupied before absorption occurs (i.e., accepted or rejected), given that the initial state is 1. The long-run absorption probability matrix, F, is calculated as follows [4],

$$F = M \times R = 1\begin{bmatrix} \frac{p_{12}}{1-p_{11}} & \frac{p_{13}}{1-p_{11}} \end{bmatrix} \tag{22}$$

(with columns labelled 2 and 3)

The elements of the F matrix, f_{12}, f_{13}, denote the probabilities of the batch being accepted or rejected, respectively.

The expected cost can be obtained using Eq. (17) containing the batch acceptance, rejection, and inspection costs. The expected acceptance cost is the cost of nonconforming items (Npc) multiplied by the probability of the batch being accepted (i.e., f_{12}). The expected rejection cost is the rejection cost (R) multiplied by the probability of the batch being rejected (i.e., f_{13}). Moreover, m_{11} is the expected long-run number of times the transient state 1 is occupied before absorption occurs. Knowing that in each visit to transient state, the average number of inspections is $\frac{1}{p}$ (the mean of the geometric distribution), the expected inspection cost is given by

$$E(I)=\frac{I}{p}m_{11} \tag{23}$$

Therefore, the expected cost for acceptance-sampling policy can be expressed as a function of f_{12}, f_{13} and m_{11} as follows:

$$E(TC)=cNpf_{12}+Rf_{13}+\frac{I}{p}m_{11} \tag{24}$$

Substituting for f_{12} and m_{11}, the expected cost equation can be rewritten as:

$$E(TC)=Npc\frac{p_{12}}{1-p_{11}}+R\left(1-\frac{p_{12}}{1-p_{11}}\right)+\frac{I}{p}\left(\frac{1}{1-p_{11}}\right) \tag{25}$$

Eq. (25) can be solved numerically using search algorithms to find L and U that minimize the expected total cost. The objective function, $E(TC)$, should be minimized regarding two constraints on Type-I and Type-II errors associated with the acceptance sampling plans. Type-I error is the probability of rejecting the batch when the nonconformity proportion of the batch is acceptable. Type-II error is the probability of accepting the batch when the nonconforming proportion of the batch is not acceptable. Then, in one hand, if $p=AQL$, the probability of rejecting the batch should be less than α. On the other hand, in case where $p=LQL$, the probability of accepting the batch should be less than β where α and β are the probabilities of Type-I and Type-II errors, hence,

$$\begin{aligned} p=AQL \quad &\rightarrow \quad \frac{\Pr\{Y_i \geq U\}}{1-\Pr\{L<Y_i<U\}} \geq 1-\alpha \\ p=LQL \quad &\rightarrow \quad 1-\frac{\Pr\{Y_i \geq U_i\}}{1-\Pr\{L<Y_i<U\}} \geq 1-\beta \end{aligned} \tag{26}$$

The optimum values of L and U among a set of alternative values are determined solving the model given in (25), numerically, where the probabilities are obtained using the geometric distribution.

4. Acceptance Sampling Policy Using the Minimum Angle Method based on Number of Successive Conforming Items [5]

The practical performance of any sampling plan is determined through its operating characteristic curve. When producer and consumer are negotiating for designing sampling plans, it is important especially to minimize the consumer risk. In order to minimize the consumer's risk, the ideal OC curve could be made to pass as closely through$[AQL, 1-\alpha]$,$[AQL, \beta]$. One approach to minimize the consumers risks for ideal condition is proposed with minimization of angle ϕ between the lines joining the points$[AQL, 1-\alpha]$, $[AQL, \beta]$and $[AQL, 1-\alpha]$,$[LQL, \beta]$. Therefore in this case, the value of performance criteria in minimum angle method will be [6],

$$Tan(\phi)=\left(\frac{LQL - AQL}{\Pr_a(AQL)-\Pr_a(LQL)}\right) \tag{27}$$

where $\Pr_a(LQL)$, $\Pr_a(AQL)$is the probability of accepting the batch when the proportion of defective items in the batch is respectivelyLQL, AQL. Assume A is the point$[AQL, 1-\alpha]$, $B$is the point $[AQL, \beta]$and C is the point $[LQL, \beta]$thus the smaller value of$Tan(\phi)$, the angle ϕ approaching zero, and the chord AC approachingAB, the ideal condition.

The values of $\Pr_a(LQL)$, $\Pr_a(AQL)$ are determined as follows,

$$\begin{aligned} p=AQL &\rightarrow \Pr_a(AQL)=f_{12}(AQL)=\frac{\Pr\{U \le Y_i\}}{1-\Pr\{U > Y_i > L\}} \\ p=LQL &\rightarrow 1-\Pr_a(LQL)=1-f_{12}(LQL)=1-\frac{\Pr\{U \le Y_i\}}{1-\Pr\{U > Y_i > L\}} \end{aligned} \tag{28}$$

Since the values of LQL, AQL are constant andLQL AQL therefore the objective function is determined as follows,

$$V=\underset{L,U}{Min}\{\Pr_a(LQL)-\Pr_a(AQL)\} \tag{29}$$

Another performance measure of acceptance sampling plans is the expected number of inspected items. Since sampling and inspecting usually has cost, therefore designs that minimizes this measure and satisfy the first and second type error inequalities are considered to be optimal sampling plans. Since the proportion of defective items is not known in the start of process, in order to consider this property in designing the acceptance sampling plans, we try to minimize the expected number of inspected items for acceptable and not acceptable lots simultaneously. Therefore the optimal acceptance sampling plan should have three properties, first it should have a minimized value in the objective function of the minimum angle method that is resulted from the ideal OC curve and also it should minimize the expected number of inspected items either in the decisions of rejecting or accepting the lot. Therefore the second objective function is defined as the expected number of items inspected. The value of this objective function is determined based on the value of$m_{11}(p)$where $m_{11}(p)$ is the expected number of times in the long run that the transient state 1 is occupied before absorption occurs, since in each visit to transient state, the average number of inspections is$\frac{1}{p}$, consequently the expected number of items inspected is given by$\frac{1}{p}m_{11}(p)$. Now the objective functions W and Z are defined as the expected number of items inspected respectively in the acceptable condition($p = AQL$) and not acceptable condition($p = LQL$).

$$W = \underset{L,U}{Min}\left\{\frac{1}{AQL}m_{11}\left(AQL\right)\right\}$$
$$Z = \underset{L,U}{Min}\left\{\frac{1}{LQL}m_{11}\left(LQL\right)\right\} \tag{30}$$

Now one approach to optimize the objective functions simultaneously is to define control thresholds for objective functions Z, W and then trying to minimize the value of objective function V. For example if parameters Z_1, W_1 are defined as the upper control thresholds for Z, W then the optimization problem can be defined as follows,

$$\begin{aligned} &\underset{L,U}{Min}\{V\} \\ &S.t. \\ &Z < Z_1, W < W_1 \end{aligned} \tag{31}$$

Optimal values of L , U can be determined by solving above nonlinear optimization problem using search procedures or other optimization tools.

5. Acceptance Sampling Policy Based on Cumulative Sum of Conforming Items Run Lengths [7]

In an acceptance-sampling plan, assume Y_i is the number of conforming items between the successive $(i-1)^{th}$ and i^{th} defective items. Decision making is based on the value of S_i that is defined as,

$$S_i = Y_i + Y_{i-1} \tag{32}$$

The proposed acceptance sampling policy is defined as follows,

If $S_i \geq U$ then the batch is accepted

If $S_i \leq L$ the batch is rejected

If $L < S_i < U$ the process of inspecting the items continues

where U is the upper control threshold and L is the lower control threshold.

In each stage of the data gathering process, the index of different states of the Markov model, j , is defined as:

$j=1$ represents the state of rejecting the batch. In this state $S_i \leq L$ thus the batch is rejected.

$j=Y_i+2$ where $Y_i=0, 1, 2..., U-1$ represents the state of continuing data gathering. In this state, $L < S_i = Y_i + Y_{i-1} < U$ thus the inspecting process continues.

$j=U+2$ represents the state of accepting the batch. In this state $S_i \geq U$ hence the batch is accepted.

In other word, the acceptance-sampling plan can be expressed by a Markov model, in which the transition probability matrix among the states of the batch can be expressed as:

$$p_{jk} = \begin{cases} 1 & j=k=1 \\ 0 & j=1, k>1 \\ \Pr(Y_{i+1} \leq L - j + 2) & U+2>j>1, L \geq j-2, k=1 \\ 0 & U+2>j>1, L<j-2, k=1 \\ 0 & U+2>j>1, U+2>k>1, j+k-4 \leq L \\ 0 & U+2>j>1, U+2>k>1, j+k-4 \geq U \\ \Pr(Y_{i+1} = k-2) & U+2>j>1, U+2>k>1, U>j+k-4>L \\ 1 & j=k=U+2 \\ 0 & j=U+2, k<U+2 \\ \Pr(Y_{i+1} \geq U - j + 2) & U+2>j>1, k=U+2 \end{cases} \tag{33}$$

where, p_{jk} is probability of going from state j to state k in a single step and Y_{i+1} denotes the number of conforming items between the successive defective items and $\Pr(Y_{i+1}=r)=(1-p)^r p \quad r=0, 1, 2, ...$ where p denotes the proportion of defective items in the batch.

The values of p_{jk} are determined based on the relations among the states, for example where $U+2>j>1$, $L \geq j-2$, $k=1$ then according to the definition of j, it is concluded that $j=Y_i+2$ and transition probability of going form state j to state $k=1$ is equal to the probability of rejecting the batch that is evaluated as follows,

$$p_{j1}=\Pr(L \geq S_{i+1}=Y_{i+1}+Y_i)=\Pr(L \geq Y_{i+1}+j-2)=\Pr(Y_{i+1} \leq L - j + 2) \tag{34}$$

In the other case where, $U+2>j>1$, $U+2>k>1$, $U>j+k-4>L$, based on the definition of j, we have $j=Y_i+2$ thus it is concluded that

$$\begin{aligned} p_{jk} &= \Pr(L < S_{i+1} = Y_{i+1} + Y_i < U,\ Y_{i+1}=k-2) = \\ &\Pr(L < j-2+Y_{i+1} < U,\ Y_{i+1}=k-2) = \\ &\Pr(L < j-2+k-2 < U,\ Y_{i+1}=k-2) = \Pr(L < j+k-4 < U,\ Y_{i+1}=k-2) \end{aligned} \tag{35}$$

In the other case where, $U+2>j>1$, $k=U+2$, then according to the definition of j, we have $j=Y_i+2$ thus it is concluded that,

$$p_{jU+2}=\Pr(S_{i+1}=Y_{i+1}+Y_i\geq U)=\Pr(Y_{i+1}+j-2\geq U)=\Pr(Y_{i+1}\geq U-j+2) \tag{36}$$

In the other case where, $U+2>j>1$, $U+2>k>1$, $j+k-4\geq U$, then according to the definition of j, we have $j=Y_i+2$ thus it is concluded that,

$$\begin{aligned} p_{jk} &= \Pr(L<S_{i+1}=Y_{i+1}+Y_i<U,\ Y_{i+1}=k-2,\ j+k-4\geq U) \\ &= \Pr(L<j-2+Y_{i+1}<U,\ Y_{i+1}=k-2,\ j+k-4\geq U) \\ &= \Pr(L<j+k-4<U,\ j+k-4\geq U)=0 \end{aligned} \tag{37}$$

As a result, when $L=1$and $U=3$ for example, the transition probability matrix among the states of the system can be expressed as:

$$\mathbf{P}=\begin{matrix} & 1 & 2 & 3 & 4 & 5 \\ 1 & 1 & 0 & 0 & 0 & 0 \\ 2 & \Pr(Y\leq 1) & 0 & 0 & \Pr(Y=2) & \Pr(Y\geq 3) \\ 3 & \Pr(Y\leq 0) & 0 & \Pr(Y=1) & 0 & \Pr(Y\geq 2) \\ 4 & 0 & \Pr(Y=0) & 0 & 0 & \Pr(Y\geq 1) \\ 5 & 0 & 0 & 0 & 0 & 1 \end{matrix} \tag{38}$$

And it can be seen the matrix $\boldsymbol{P}$ is an absorbing Markov chain with states 1 and 5 being absorbing and states 2, 3, and 4 being transient.

Analyzing the above absorbing Markov chain requires to rearrange the single-step probability matrix in the following form:

$$P=\begin{bmatrix} \boldsymbol{A} & \boldsymbol{O} \\ \boldsymbol{R} & \boldsymbol{Q} \end{bmatrix} \tag{39}$$

where$A$is the identity matrix representing the probability of staying in a state that is defined as follows

$$A=\begin{bmatrix} 1 & 0 \\ 0 & 1 \end{bmatrix} \tag{40}$$

$\boldsymbol{O}$is the probability matrix of escaping an absorbing state (always zero) that is defined as follows

$$O = \begin{array}{c} \\ 1 \\ 5 \end{array} \begin{array}{c} \begin{array}{ccc} 2 & 3 & 4 \end{array} \\ \begin{bmatrix} 0 & 0 & 0 \\ 0 & 0 & 0 \end{bmatrix} \end{array} \tag{41}$$

Q is a square matrix containing the transition probabilities of going from a non-absorbing state to another non-absorbing state that is defined as follows

$$Q = \begin{array}{c|ccc} & 2 & 3 & 4 \\ \hline 2 & 0 & 0 & \Pr(Y=2) \\ 3 & 0 & \Pr(Y=1) & 0 \\ 4 & \Pr(Y=0) & 0 & 0 \end{array} \tag{42}$$

And $R$is the Matrix containing all probabilities of going from a non-absorbing state to an absorbing state (i.e., accepted or rejected batch) that is defined as follows

$$\mathbf{R} = \begin{array}{c|cc} & 1 & 5 \\ \hline 2 & \Pr(Y \le 1) & \Pr(Y \ge 3) \\ 3 & \Pr(Y \le 0) & \Pr(Y \ge 2) \\ 4 & 0 & \Pr(Y \ge 1) \end{array} \tag{43}$$

Rearranging the P matrix in the latter form yields the following:

$$\mathbf{P} = \begin{array}{c|ccccc} & 1 & 5 & 2 & 3 & 4 \\ \hline 1 & 1 & 0 & 0 & 0 & 0 \\ 5 & 0 & 1 & 0 & 0 & 0 \\ 2 & \Pr(Y \le 1) & \Pr(Y \ge 3) & 0 & 0 & \Pr(Y=2) \\ 3 & \Pr(Y \le 0) & \Pr(Y \ge 2) & 0 & \Pr(Y=1) & 0 \\ 4 & 0 & \Pr(Y \ge 1) & \Pr(Y=0) & 0 & 0 \end{array} \tag{44}$$

Bowling et. al. [4] proposed an absorbing Markov chain model for determining the optimal process means. According to their method, matrix Mthat is the fundamental matrix containing the expected number of transitions from a non-absorbing state to another non-absorbing state before absorption occurs can be obtained by the following equation,

$$M = (I - Q)^{-1} \tag{45}$$

For the above numerical example, i.e., when $L = 1$and$U = 3$, the fundamental matrix M can be obtained as:

$$\mathbf{M}=(\mathbf{I}-\mathbf{Q})^{-1}=\begin{matrix} 2\\3\\4\end{matrix}\begin{bmatrix} \overset{2}{1} & \overset{3}{0} & \overset{4}{-\Pr(Y=2)} \\ 0 & 1-\Pr(Y=1) & 0 \\ -\Pr(Y=0) & 0 & 1 \end{bmatrix}^{-1} \tag{46}$$

where I is the identity matrix.

Since m_{jj} represents the expected number of the times in the long-run the transient state j is occupied before absorption occurs (i.e., before accepted or rejected), and matrix F is the absorption probability matrix containing the long run probabilities of the transition from a non-absorbing state to an absorbing state. The long-run absorption probability matrix, F, can be calculated as follows:

$$F=M\times R \tag{47}$$

Again when $L=1$ and $U=3$, the elements of F $(f_{jk}\ ;\ j=2,3,4\ ;\ k=1,5)$ represent the probabilities of the batch being accepted and rejected, respectively, given that the initial state is $j=2, 3, 4$. In this case, the probability of accepting the batch is obtained as:

$$\begin{aligned}&\text{Probability of accepting the batch}=\\&\sum_{j=2}^{\infty}\Pr(\text{Accepting the batch} \mid \text{the initial state is } j)\times\Pr(\text{the initial state is } j)\\&=\sum_{j=2}^{4} f_{j5}\Pr(Y=j-2)+\Pr(Y\geq 3)\end{aligned} \tag{48}$$

Also the expected number of inspected items will be determined as follows,

$$\begin{aligned}&\text{Expected number of inspected items}=\\&\sum_{j=2}^{U+1}\begin{pmatrix}\text{(the number of inspected items in state j)}\\\text{(the number of visits to state j)}\end{pmatrix}=\sum_{j=2}^{U+1}(j-2)m_{jj}\end{aligned} \tag{49}$$

This new acceptance-sampling plan should satisfy two constraints of the first and the second types of errors. The probability of Type-I error shows the probability of rejecting the batch when the defective proportion of the batch is acceptable. The probability of Type-II error is the probability of accepting the batch when the defective proportion of the batch is not acceptable. Then on the one hand if $p=AQL$, the probability of rejecting the batch will be less than α and on the other hand, in case where $p=LQL$, the probability of accepting the batch will be less than β where α and β are the probabilities of Type-I and Type-II errors. Hence,

$$
\begin{aligned}
&p = AQL \rightarrow \text{Probability of accepting the batch} \geq 1-\alpha \\
&p = LQL \rightarrow \text{Probability of accepting the batch} \leq \beta
\end{aligned}
\tag{50}
$$

From the inequalities in (50), the proper values of the thresholds L and U are determined and among the feasible ones, we select one that has the least value for [illegible] inspected items that is obtained using Eq. (49).

6. A New Acceptance Sampling Design Using Bayesian Modelling and Backwards Induction [8]

In this research, a new selection approach on the choices between accepting and rejecting a batch based on Bayesian modelling and backwards induction is proposed. The Bayesian modelling is utilized to model the uncertainty involved in the probability distribution of the nonconforming proportion of the items and the backwards induction method is employed to determine the sample size. Moreover, when the decision on accepting or rejecting a batch cannot be made, we assume additional observations can be gathered with a cost to update the probability distribution of the nonconforming proportion of the batch. In other words, a mathematical model is developed in this research to design optimal single sampling plans. This model finds the optimum sampling design whereas its optimality is resulted by using the decision tree approach. As a result, the main contribution of the method is to model the acceptance-sampling problem as a cost optimization model so that the optimal solution can be achieved via using the decision tree approach. In this approach, the required probabilities of decision tree are determined employing the Bayesian Inference. To do this, the probability distribution function of nonconforming proportion of items is first determined by Bayesian inference using a non-informative prior distribution. Then, the required probabilities are determined by applying Bayesian inference in the backward induction method of the decision tree approach. Since this model is completely designed based on the Bayesian inference and no approximation is needed, it can be viewed as a new tool to be used by practitioners in real case problems to design an economically optimal acceptance-sampling plan. However, the main limitation of the proposed methodology is that it can only be applied to items not requiring very low fractions of nonconformities.

6.1. Notations

The following notations are used throughout the paper.

Set of decisions: $A = \{a_1, a_2\}$is defined the set of possible decisions where a_1 and a_2 refer to accepting and rejecting the batch, respectively.

State space: $P = \{p_l;\ l = 1, 2, \ldots;\ 0 < p_l < 1\}$is defined the state of the process where $p_l$represents nonconforming proportion items of the batch in l^{th} state of the process. The decision maker believes the consequences of selecting decisiona_1 or a_2 depend on P that cannot be determined with certainty. However, the probability distribution function of the random variable p can be obtained using Bayesian inference.

Set of experiments: $E=\{e_i; i=1, 2, ...\}$is the set of experiments to gather more information on $p$and consequently to update the probability distribution of$p$. Further, $e_i$is defined an experiment in which $i$items of the batch are inspected.

Sample space: $Z=\{z_j; j=0, 1, 2, ..., i\}$denotes the outcomes of experiment e_i where $z_j$shows the number of nonconforming items ine_i.

Cost function: The function $u(e, z, a, p)$ on $E\times Z\times A\times P$ denotes the cost associated with performing experiment$e$, observing$z$, making decision$a$, and finding$p$.

N: The total number of items in a batch

R: The cost of rejecting a batch

C: The cost of one nonconforming item

S: The cost of inspecting one item

n: An upper bound on the number of inspected item

6.2. Problem Definition

Consider a batch of size N with an unknown percentage of nonconforming p and assume m items are randomly selected for inspection. Based on the outcome of the inspection process in terms of the observed number of nonconforming items, the decision-maker desires to accept the batch, reject it, or to perform more inspections by taking more samples. As Raiffa & Schlaifer [9] stated "the problem is how the decision maker chose $e$and then, having observed$z$, choose $e$such that $u(e, z, a, p)$ is minimized. Although the decision maker has full control over his choice of $e$and$a$, he has neither control over the choices of $z$nor$p$. However, we can assume he is able to assign probability distribution function over these choices." They formulated this problem in the framework of the decision tree approach, the one that is partially adapted in this research as well.

6.3. Bayesian Modelling

For a nonconforming proportion$p$, referring to Jeffrey's prior (Nair et al. [10]), we first take a Beta prior distribution with parameters v_0=0.5 and u_0=0.5 to model the absolute uncertainty. Then, the posterior probability density function of p using a sample of $v+u$ inspected items is

$$f(p)=Beta(v+0.5,\ u+0.5)=\frac{\Gamma(v+u+1)}{\Gamma(v+0.5)\Gamma(u+0.5)}p^{v-0.5}(1-p)^{u-0.5} \tag{51}$$

where v is the number of nonconforming items and u is the number of conforming items in the sample. Moreover, to allow more flexibility in representing prior uncertainty it is convenient to define a discrete distribution by discretization of the Beta density (Mazzuchi, & Soyer [11]) In other words, we define the prior distribution for p_l as

$$\Pr\{p=p_l\}=\int_{p_1-\delta/2}^{p_1+\delta/2} f(p)dp \tag{52}$$

where $p_1=\left(\frac{2l-1}{2}\right)\delta$ and $\delta=\frac{1}{m}$ for $l=1, 2, ..., m$

Now, define $(j, i); i=1, 2, ..., n$ and $j=0, 1, 2, ..., i$ the experiment in which j nonconforming items are found when i items are inspected. Then, the sample space Z becomes $Z=\{(j, i): 0\leq j\leq i\leq n\}$, resulting in the cost function representation of $u[e_i, (j, i), a_k, p_1]; k=1, 2$ that is associated with taking a sample of i items, observing j nonconforming and adopting a_1 or a_2 when the defective proportion is p_l. Using the notations defined, the cost function is determined by the following equations:

$$\begin{aligned}&\text{1) for accepted batch}\\&u(e_i, (j, i), a_1, p_1)=CN\,p_1+Se_i\\&\text{2) for rejected batch}\\&u(e_i, (j, i), a_2, p_1)=R+Se_i\end{aligned} \tag{53}$$

Moreover, the probability of finding j nonconforming items in a sample of i inspected items, i.e., $\Pr\{(j, i)\mid p=p_1\}$, can be obtained using a binomial distribution with parameters $(i, p=p_l)$ as:

$$\Pr\{(j, i)\mid p=p_1\}=C_j^i\,p_1^j(1-p_1)^{i-j} \tag{54}$$

Hence, the probability $\Pr\{p=p_1, z=z_j\mid e=e_i\}$ can be calculated as follows

$$\begin{aligned}\Pr\{p=p_1, z=z_j\mid e=e_i\}&=\Pr\{z=z_j\mid p=p_1, e=e_i\}\Pr\{p=p_1\}\\&=C_j^i\,p_1^j(1-p_1)^{i-j}\int_{p_1-\delta/2}^{p_1+\delta/2} f(p)dp\end{aligned} \tag{55}$$

Thus,

$$\Pr\{z=z_j \mid e=e_i\}=\sum_{l=1}^{m}\Pr\{p=p_l,\ z=z_j \mid e=e_i\}\Pr\{p=p_l\}$$
$$=\sum_{l=1}^{m}\left(C_j^i p_1^j(1-p_1)^{i-j}\int_{p_1-\delta/2}^{p_1+\delta/2} f(p)dp\right) \tag{56}$$

In other words, applying the Bayesian rule, the probability $\Pr\{p=p_l \mid z=z_j,\ e=e_i\}$ can be obtained by

$$\Pr\{p=p_1 \mid z=z_j,\ e=e_i\}=\frac{\Pr\{p=p_1,\ z=z_j \mid e=e_i\}}{\Pr\{z=z_j \mid e=e_i\}}$$
$$=\frac{C_j^i p_1^j(1-p_1)^{i-j}\int_{p_1-\delta/2}^{p_1+\delta/2} f(p)dp}{\sum_{k=1}^{m} C_j^i p_k^j(1-p_k)^{i-j}\int_{p_k-\delta/2}^{p_k+\delta/2} f(p)dp} \tag{57}$$

In the next Section, a backward induction approach is taken to determine the optimal sample size.

6.4. Backward Induction

The analysis continues by working backwards from the terminal decisions of the decision tree to the base of the tree, instead of starting by asking which experiment $e$the decision maker should select when he does not know the outcomes of the random events. This method of working back from the outermost branches of the decision tree to the initial starting point is often called "backwards induction" [9]. As a result, the steps involved in the solution algorithm of the problem at hand using the backwards induction becomes

1. Probabilities $\Pr\{p=p_l\}$ and $\Pr\{(j,\ i) \mid p=p_l\}$ are determined using Eq. (52) and Eq. (54), respectively.

2. The conditional probability $\Pr\{p=p_l \mid z=z_j,\ e=e_i\}$ is determined using Eq. (57).

3. With a known history$(e,\ z)$, since $p$is a random variable, the costs of various possible terminal decisions are uncertain. Therefore the cost of any decision a for the given $(e,\ z)$ is set as a random variable$u(e,\ z,\ a,\ p)$. Applying the conditional expectation, $E_{p \mid z}$, which takes the expected value of $u(e,\ z,\ a,\ p)$ with respect to the conditional probability $P_{p \mid z}$(Eq. 57), the conditional expected value of the cost function on state variable p_1 is determined by the following equation.

$$u^*(e_i, z_j, a_k) = \sum_{l=1}^{m} (u^*(e_i, z_j, a_k, p_1) \Pr\{p = p_1 \mid z = z_j, e = e_i\}) \tag{58}$$

4. Since the objective is to minimize the expected cost, the cost of having history (e, z) and the choice of decision (accepting or rejecting) can be determined by

$$u^*(e_i, z_j) = \min_{a_k} u^*(e_i, z_j, a_k) \tag{59}$$

5. The conditional probability $\Pr\{z = z_j \mid e = e_i\}$ is determined using Eq. (56).

6. The costs of various possible experiments are random because the outcome $z$is a random variable. Defining a probability distribution function over the results of experiments and taking expected values, we can determine the expected cost of each experiment. The conditional expected value of function $u^*(e_i, z_j)$ on the variable z_j is determined by the following equation.

$$u^*(e_i) = \sum_{j=0}^{i} \{u^*(e_i, z_j) \Pr\{z = z_j \mid e = e_i\}\} \tag{60}$$

7. Now the minimum of the values $u^*(e_i)$ would be the optimal decision, which leads to an optimal sample size.

$$u^* = \min_e u^*(e_i) = \min_e E_{z \mid e} \min_a E_{p \mid z} u(e_i, z_j, a_k, p_1) \tag{61}$$

7. Conclusion

Acceptance sampling plans have been widely used in industry to determine whether a specific batch of manufactured or purchased items satisfy a pre-specified quality. In this chapter, new models for determining optimal acceptance sampling plans have been presented. The relationship between the cost model and a decision theory model with probabilistic utilities has been investigated. However, the acceptance sampling plan, which are derived from the optimization of these models, may differ substantially from the plans that other economic approaches suggest but optimization of these models are simple and efficient, with negligible computational requirements. In next sections, a new methodology based on Markov chain was developed to design proper lot acceptance sampling plans. In the proposed procedure, the sum of two successive numbers of nonconforming items was monitored using two lower and upper thresholds, where the proper values of these thresholds could be determined numerically using a Markovian approach based on the two points on OC curve. In last section, based on the Bayesian modelling and the backwards induction method of the decision-tree approach, a sampling plan is developed to deal with the lot-sentencing problem; aiming to determine an optimal sample size to provide desired levels of protection for customers as well as manufacturers. A logical analysis of the choices between accepting and rejecting a batch is made when the distribution function of nonconforming proportion could be updated by taking additional observations and using Bayesian modelling.

Author details

Mohammad Saber Fallah Nezhad*

Address all correspondence to: Fallahnezhad@yazduni.ac.ir

Assistant Professor of Industrial Engineering, Yazd University, Iran

References

[1] Fallahnezhad, M. S., & Hosseininasab, H. (2011). Designing a Single Stage Acceptance Sampling Plan based on the control Threshold policy. *International Journal of Industrial Engineering & Production Research*, 22(3), 143-150.

[2] Hilbe, J. M. (2007). Negative Binomial Regression. Cambridge, UK, : Cambridge University Press.

[3] Fallahnezhad, M. S., & Niaki, S. T. A. (2011). A New Acceptance Sampling Policy Based on Number of Successive Conforming Items. *To Appear in Communications in Statistics-Theory and Methods.*

[4] Bowling, S. R., Khasawneh, M. T., Kaewkuekool, S., & Cho, B. R. (2004). A Markovian approach to determining optimum process target levels for a multi-stage serial production system. *European Journal of Operational Research*, 159-636.

[5] Fallahnezhad, M. S. (2012). A New Approach for Acceptance Sampling Policy Based on the Number of Successive Conforming Items and Minimum Angle Method. *To Appear in Iranian Journal of Operations Research.*, 3(1), 104-111.

[6] Soundararajan, V., & Christina, A. L. (1997). Selection of single sampling variables plans based on the minimum angle. *Journal of Applied Statistics*, 24(2), 207-218.

[7] Fallahnezhad, M. S., Niaki, S. T. A., & Abooie, M. H. (2011). A New Acceptance Sampling Plan Based on Cumulative Sums of Conforming Run-Lengths. *Journal of Industrial and Systems Engineering*, 4(4), 256-264.

[8] Fallahnezhad, M. S., Niaki, S. T. A., & Vahdat, M. A. (2012). A New Acceptance Sampling Design Using Bayesian Modeling and Backwards Induction. *International Journal of Engineering, Islamic Republic of Iran*, 25(1), 45-54.

[9] Raiffa, H. (2000). Schlaifer R. Applied statistical decision theory. New York, Wiley Classical Library.

[10] Nair, V. N., Tang, B., & Xu, L. (2001). Bayesian inference for some mixture problems in quality and reliability. *Journal of Quality Technology*, 33-16.

[11] Mazzuchi, T. A., & Soyer, R. (1996). Adaptive Bayesian replacement strategies. Pro- [illegible] Ber- nardo, J. O. Berger, A. P. Dawid, and A. F. M. Smith, eds.)Elsevier , 667-674.

Chapter 3

Applications of Control Charts Arima for Autocorrelated Data

Suzana Leitão Russo, Maria Emilia Camargo and Jonas Pedro Fabris

Additional information is available at the end of the chapter

1. Introduction

The traditional methodology of Statistical Quality Control (SEQ) is based on a fundamental supposition that the process of the data is independent statisticaly, however, the data not always are independent. When a process follows an adaptable model, or when the process is a deterministic function, the data will be autocorrelated.

Drawing the process of data is extremely valuable, however, under such circumstances, there isn't any scientific reason to use the traditional techniques of statistical control of quality, because it will induce erroneous conclusions and facilitate a safety absence that the process is under statistical control with flaw in the identification of systematic variation of the process.

Thus, the theme here proposed is to investigate the acting and the adaptation of the traditional use of the statistical control of process methods in no-stationary processes, and to discuss the use of time series methodologies to work with correlated observations.

2. Theorical Review

History of Quality Control is as old as the history of the industry itself. Before the Industrial Revolution, the quality was controlled by the vast experience of the artisans of the time, which guarantee product quality. The industrial system has suffered a new technical era, where the production process split complex operations into simple tasks that could be performed by workers with specific skills. Thus, the worker is no longer responsible for all product manufacturing, leaving the responsibility of only a part of it (Juran, 1993).

It is within this context that the inspection, which sought to separate the non-conforming items from the establishment of specifications and tolerances. A simple inspection did not improve the quality of products, only provided information on the quality level of these and pick the items conform, those not complying. The constant concern with costs and productivity has led to the question: how to use information obtained through inspection to improve the quality of products?

The solution of this question led to the recognition that variability was a factor inherent in industrial processes and could be understood through the statistics and probability, noting that could be measurements made during the manufacturing process without having to wait for the completion of the production cycle.

In 1924, Dr. Walter. A. Shewhart of Bell Telephone Laboratories, developed a statistical graph to monitor and control the production process, being one of the tools of Statistical Quality Control. The purpose of these graphs was differentiate between aleatórias1 causes unavoidable and causes a remarkable process. According to Shewhart (1931), if the random causes were present, one should not tamper with the process, if assignable causes are present, one should detect them and eliminate them. In other words, these graphics monitor the change or lack of instability in the process thus ensuring quality products.

Studies by Johnson and Basgshaw (1974) and Harris and Ross (1991) showed that the graphics Shewhart and cumulative sums (CUSUM) are sensitive to the presence of autocorrelated data (data that are not independent of each other over time), especially when the autocorrelation is extreme, ie tools are not suitable for the process control.

You will need to process the data first and then control them statistically. The presence of autocorrelation in the data leads to growth in the number of false alarms. Alwan and Roberts (1988) show that many false alarms (signals of special causes) may occur in the presence of moderate levels of autocorrelation, and the resulting measurement system, the dynamics of the process or both aspects, and conventional control charts are used without knowing the presence or absence of correlation, much effort can be spent in vain.

Many methods have been proposed to deal with statistical data autocorrelation. The interest in the area was stimulated by the work of Box and Jenkins, published in 1970 work entitled Time Series Analysis: Forecasting and Control, where it was presented among several quantitative methods, methodology used to analyze the behavior of the time series. The method of Box and Jenkins uses the concept of filter composed of three components: component autoregressive (AR), the integration filter (I) component and the moving average (MA).

The reason for monitoring residual processes is that they are independent and identically distributed with mean zero, when the process is controlled and remains independent of possible differences in the mean when the process gets out of control. Zhang (1998), the traditional graphics Shewhart, CUSUM graphics, the graphics may be applied to the EWMA waste, since the use of graphics residual control has the advantage that they can be applied to autocorrelated data, even if the data is nonstationary processes. When a graph of residual control is applied to a non stationary, it can only be concluded that the process has some deviation in the system because of a non stationary there is no constant average and / or constant variance.

3. Statistical Quality Control

The statistical quality control (SQC) is a technique of analyzing the process, setting standards, comparing performance, verify and study deviations, to seek and implement solutions, analyze the process again after the changes, seeking the best performance of machinery and / or persons (Montgomery, 1997).

Another definition is given by Triola (1999), which states that the SQC is a preventive method where the results are compared continuously through statistical data, identifying trends for significant changes, and eliminating or controlling these changes in order to reduce them more and more.

SPC charts are designed to detect shifts among natural fluctuations caused by chance noises. For example, the Shewhart chart utilizes the standard deviation (SD) statistic to measure the size of the in-control process variability. By graphically contrasting the observed deviations against a multiple (usually, triple) of SDs, the control chart is intended to identify unusual departures of the process from its normal state (controlled state).

Under certain assumptions, when the observed deviation from the mean exceeds three SDs, it is said that the process is out of control since there is only a probability of 0.0026 for the observation to fall outside the three SD limits given an unshifted mean chance the process mean is shifted. This Shewhart chart scheme is in effect a statistical hypothesis testing that reveals only whether the process is still in-control (Chen and Elsayed, 2000).

To better understand the technical statistical quality control, it is necessary to bear in mind that the quality of a product manufactured by a process is inevitably subject to variation, and which can be described in terms of two types concerned.

The *special cause* is a factor that generates variations that affect the process behavior in unpredictable ways, it is therefore possible to obtain a standard or a probability distribution.

The *common cause* is defined as a source of variation that affects all the individual values of a process. It results from various sources, without having any predominance over the other.

When these variations are significant in relation to the specifications, it runs the risk of having non-compliant products, ie products that do not meet specifications. The elimination of requiring special causes a local action, which can be made by people close to the process, for example, workers. Since the common causes require actions on the system of work that can only be taken by the administration, since the process is itself consistent, but still unable to meet specifications (Ramos, 2000).

According to Woodall et al (2004), Statistical Quality Control is a collection of tools that are essential in quality improvement activities.

Descriptive Statistics

According to Reid and Sanders (2002), descriptive statistics can be helpful in describing certain characteristics of a product and a process. The most important descriptive statistics are measures of central tendency such as the mean, measures of variability such as the standard deviation and range, and measures of the distribution of data. We first review these descriptive statistics and then see how we can measure their changes.

The mean: To compute the mean we simply sum all the observations and divide by the total number of observations. The equation for computing the mean is:

$$\bar{x} = \frac{\sum_{i=1}^{n} x_i}{n}$$

where: $\bar{x}$= mean;

x_i= the observation $i, i = 1, 2, \ldots, n$;

n= number of observation.

The range and standard deviation: There are two measures that can be used to determine the amount of variation in the data. The first measure is the *range*, which is the difference between the largest and smallest observations in a set of data. Another measure of variation is the *standard deviation*. *Standard deviation* is a statistic that measures the amount of data dispersion around the mean.The equation for computing the standard deviation is (Reid and Sanders, 2002),:

$$\sigma = \sqrt{\frac{\sum_{i-1}^{n} (x_i - \bar{x})^2}{n-1}}$$

where: σ= standard deviation of a sample

$\bar{x}$= the mean;

x_i= the observation $i, i = 1, 2, \ldots, n$;

n= number of observation in the sample

Small values of the range and standard deviation mean that the observations are closely clustered around the mean. Large values of the range and standard deviation mean that the observations are spread out around the mean.

Distribution of the data

A third descriptive statistic used to measure quality characteristics is the shape of the distribution of the observed data. When a distribution is symmetric, there are the same number of observations below and above the mean. This is what we commonly find when only normal variation is present in the data. When a disproportionate number of observations are either above or below the mean, we say that the data has a skewed distribution.

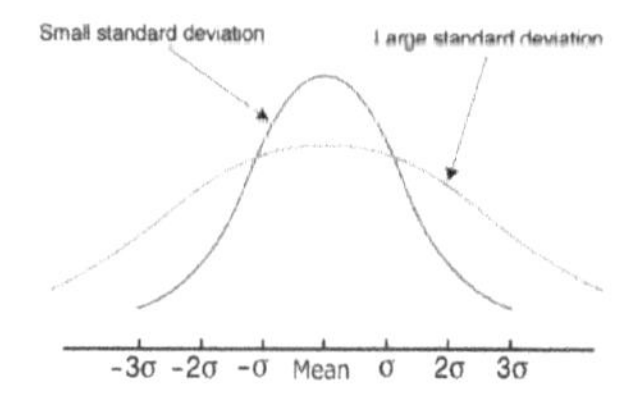

Figure 1. Normal distributions with varying standard deviations (adapted of Reid and Sanders, 2002).

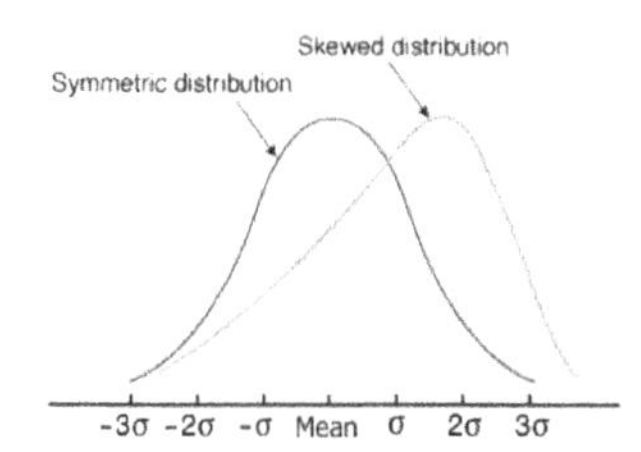

Figure 2. Differences between symmetric and skewed distributions (adapted of Reid and Sanders, 2002).

Control Charts

In any production process, no matter how well designed or carefully maintained it is, a certain amount of inherent or natural variability will always exist. Natural variability is the cumulative effect of many causes small, essentially unavoidable. When this variation is relatively small, generally considered an acceptable level of performance of the process. In the context of statistical quality control, this natural variability often called "a stable system of special causes" is said to be in statistical control. Control charts are used to examine whether or not the process is under control, ie, indicate only random causes are acting on this process. Synthesize a wide range of data using statistical methods to observe the variability within the process, based on sampling data. Can inform us at any given time as the process is behaving, if it is within prescribed limits, signaling thus the need to seek the cause of variation, but not showing us how to eliminate it (Ryan, 1989).

It was W. A. Shewhart (1931) which introduced control charts in 1924 with the intention to eliminate variations to distinguish them from the common causes and special causes. A control chart consists of three parallel lines: a line that reflects the average level of process operation, and two external lines called upper control limit (UCL) and lower control limit (LCL), calculated according to the standard deviation of a process variable (Shewhart, 1931).

There are several types of control charts, as the characteristic values or purpose, and we can divide them by attribute control charts and control charts for each variable.

Control charts by attributes

A control chart for attributes, on the other hand, is used to monitor characteristics that have discrete values and can be counted. Often they can be evaluated with a simple yes or no decision (Reid and Sanders, 2002).

There are two broad categories of control charts for attributes: those who classify items into compliance or non-compliant, as is the case of graphs of the fraction of the number of faulty or defective, and those who consider the number (amount) of nonconformity existing graphics such as the number of defects in the sample or per unit.

According to Ramos (2000), the difficulties are:

a) due to the small size of the batch, the approximation of binomial and Poisson by the normal distribution may no longer be valid, in which case the limits of control charts can not be determined by standard formulas;

b) the probability distributions Binomial and Poisson may not adequately represent the studied phenomenon. This occurs when the parts are manufactured simultaneously (multiple mold cavities, for example), in which the incidence of defects or defects is not independent, statistically speaking.

Control charts for variable

Control charts for variables monitor characteristics that can be measured and have a continuous scale, such as height, weight, volume, or width. When an item is inspected, the variable being monitored is measured and recorded (Reid and Sanders, 2002).

They may not be used for quality characteristics that cannot be measured because the control of the process requires monitoring of the mean and variability of measures. The graphics control variables used to data that can be measured or which undergo a continuous variation.

Some of the methods suitable for the construction of different control charts are the *Shewhart chart, Chart MOSUM - Moving Sum,* the *EWMA Chart - Weight Exponential Moving Average (Exponentially Weighted Moving Averages)* and *CUSUM Chart - Cumulative Sum (Cumulative Sum).*

Shewhart control charts

The first formal model of control chart was proposed by Dr. Walter A. Shewhart (1931), which now bears his name. Let X a statistical sample which measures a characteristic of the process used to control a production line. Suppose that μ is the population mean of X and σ is the population standard deviation.

The following equations are used to describe the three parameters that characterize the Shewhart control charts (Montgomery, 1997)

$$UCL = \mu + k\sigma_{\bar{x}} \quad (1)$$

$$CL = \mu \quad (2)$$

$$LCL = \mu - k\sigma_{\bar{x}} \quad (3)$$

where UCL is the upper control limit, CL is the center line or the average of the process, LCL is the lower control limit of the process, and k is the distance the control limits by the center line, which is expressed as a multiple of the σstandard deviation. The value of k is 3 most widely used.

The control graph is divided into zones (Figure 3). If a data point falls outside the control limits, we assume that the process is probably out of control and that an investigation is warranted to find and eliminate the cause or causes.

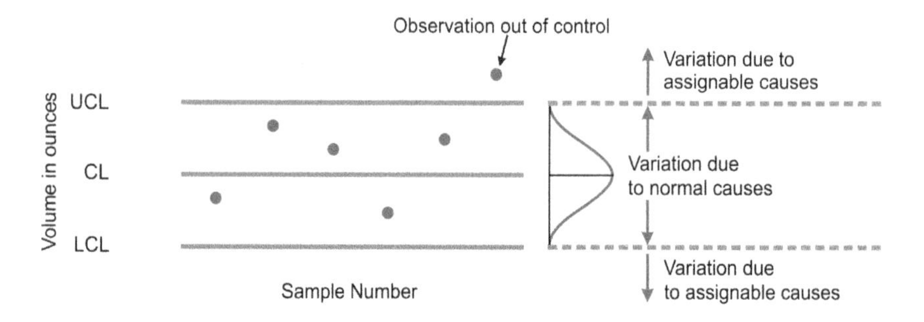

Figure 3. Control chart (adapted of Reid and Sanders, 2002).

$\overline{X}$ - S Control Charts

A mean control chart is often referred to as an $\overline{X}$chart. It is used to monitor changes in the mean of a process. The $\overline{X}$ - S control charts are generally preferred over the $\overline{X}$ - Rcharts when n10 or 12, since for larger samples the amplitude sampling R loses the efficiency to estimateσ, when compared to the sample standard deviation. The $\overline{X}$ control charts is used in order to control the mean of the considered process. The two charts should be used simultaneously (Werkema, 1995).

The limits of the $\overline{X}$ - S control charts are obtained in a similar manner, calculated under the assumption that the quality feature of interest (x) has a normal distribution with (μ) mean and (σ) standard deviation, ie, in abbreviated form (Panagiotidou and Nenes, 2009; Werkema, 1995).

$x \sim N(\mu, \sigma)$

However, satisfactory results are obtained even when this assumption is not true and distribution of x can only be considered approximately normal. In practice the μ and σ parameters are unknown and must be estimated from sample data. The method of estimation of μ

and σ again involves taking m samples (subgroups rational) primary, each containing n observations of the quality characteristic considered.

Estimation of μ:

The (μ) mean is estimate through the overall average of the sample ($\bar{\bar{x}}$)as defined in the equation:

$$\bar{\bar{x}} = \frac{\bar{x}_1 + \bar{x}_2 + ... + \bar{x}_m}{m} = \frac{1}{m}\sum_{i=1}^{m} \bar{x}_i \tag{4}$$

where $\bar{x}_i$, $i = 1,2,...,m$ is the i-ésima sample mean:

$$\bar{x}_i = \frac{x_{i1} + x_{i2} + ... + x_{in}}{n} \tag{5}$$

Estimation of σ based on sample standard deviation:

The (σ) standard deviation is estimate based in the ($\bar{s}$) standard deviation mean as defined by:

$$\bar{s} = \frac{s_1 + s_2 + ... + s_m}{m} = \frac{1}{m}\sum_{i=1}^{m} s_i \tag{6}$$

where s_i, $i = 1,2,...,m$ is the i-ésima sample of the standard deviation:

$$s_i = \sqrt{\frac{1}{n-1}\sum_{l=1}^{n} (x_{ij} - \bar{x}_i)^2} \tag{7}$$

It can be shown that the standard deviation sigma must be estimated by $\hat{\sigma} = \frac{\bar{s}}{c_4}$, where c_4 is a correction factor, tabulated as a function of size n of each sample.

Expressions for calculating the limits of $\overline{X} - S$ control charts:

$\overline{X}$ control charts -

$$UCL = \bar{\bar{x}} + 3\bar{s} / c_4\sqrt{n} = \bar{\bar{x}} + A_3\bar{s} \tag{8}$$

$$CL = \bar{\bar{x}} \tag{9}$$

$$LCL = \bar{\bar{x}} - 3\bar{s} / c_4\sqrt{n} = \bar{\bar{x}} - A_3\bar{s} \tag{10}$$

where $A_3 = 3 / c_4\sqrt{n}$ is a constant tabulated as a function of size n of each sample.

S control charts -

$$UCL = \bar{s} + 3\hat{\sigma}_s = B_4\bar{s} \tag{11}$$

$$CL = \bar{s} \tag{12}$$

$$LCL = \bar{s} - 3\hat{\sigma}_s = B_3\bar{s} \tag{13}$$

where $\hat{\sigma}_s$ is a estimative of the standard deviation of the distribution of the S and B_3 and B_4 are constants tabulated in function of size n of each sample (Panagiotidou and Nenes, 2009; Werkema, 1995).

Identification of Process in Control

It is understood that the process is controlled to:

a) all points on the chart are within the control limits;

b) the arrangement of points within the control limits is random.

Identification of Process out of Control

According Montgomery (2009), various criteria may be simultaneously applied to a control graph for determining whether the process is under control. The basic criterion is one or more points outside the control limits. The additional criteria are sometimes used to increase the sensitivity of the control graphs when there is a small change in the process, so as to respond quickly to an assignable cause.

The Shewhart control charts have some rules sensitizers (Montgomery, 2009):

1. One or more points outside the control limits;
2. Two or three consecutive points outside the warning limits of 2-sigma;
3. Four or five consecutive points above of the limits of one-sigma;
4. A sequence of eight consecutive points of a same side of the center line;
5. Six points in a sequence is always increasing or decreasing;
6. Fifteen points in sequence in the area C (both above and below the center line);
7. Fourteen points alternately in sequence up or down;
8. Sequence of eight points on both sides of the center line CL;
9. A standard non-random data;
10. One or more points near a limit or control.

Typical patterns of behavior are non-random (Lourenço Filho, 1964):

a) *Periodicity* - increases and decreases at regular intervals of time. The periodicity appears as one of the operating conditions of the process suffers periodic changes or when regular exchange of machines or operators.

b) *Trend* - when the points are directed substantially upwards, or downwards. The general trend indicates a gradual deterioration of a critical process. This "decay" can be a tool wear and operator fatigue.

c) *Shift* - changes in performance of the process. The cause of the change can be introduction of new machinery, new operators, new methods or even a quality program, which usually brings motivation and improves performance.

4. Time Series

The time series analysis aims to: investigate the mechanism generating the time series; to forecast future values of the series, to describe the behavior of the series; seek relevant periodicities in the data. A model that describes a series does not necessarily lead to a procedure (or formula) prediction. You need to specify a function-loss, beyond the model, to get the procedure. A function-loss, which is often used, is the mean square error, although on some occasions, other criteria or loss functions are more appropriate (Morettin and Toloi, 2006; Camargo and Russo, 2011).

Autocorrelation

The autocorrelation is a measure of dependency between observations Same series separated by a given range named retardation.

Be a time seriesY_t. The ratio between the covariance (Y_t, Y_{t-k}) and variance (Y_t) defines a autocorrelation coefficient simple (r_k), while the sequence of $r_k$values is called autocorrelation function simple (AFS) (Camargo and Russo, 2006).

The graphical representation of this function is called correlogram. Formally, the autocorrelation coefficients simple between Y_t and their Y_{t-k}lagged values, are defined by:

$$r_k = \frac{\text{cov}(Y_t, Y_{t-k})}{\text{var}(Y_t)} = \frac{\sum_{t=k+1}^{n} (Y_t - \bar{Y})(Y_{t-k} - \bar{Y})}{\sum_{t=1}^{n} (Y_t - \bar{Y})^2} \quad (14)$$

We can see the existence of unit root if the values of the autocorrelation function begin near to unit and decline slowly and gradually as increases the distance (number of lags, k) between the two sets of observations to which they concern, calling himself, not stationary and follows a random walk. If these coefficients decline rapidly as this distance increases, there is a series of characteristics of stationary (Morettin and Toloi, 2006; Russo et al. 2006).

Stationary Processes

A common assumption in many time series techniques is that the data are stationary. A stationary process has the property that the mean, variance and autocorrelation structure do not change over time. A process is considered stationary if its statistical characteristics do not change with time.

Stationarity is a assumption in time series analysis. It means that the main statistical properties of the series remain unchanged over time. More precisely, a process $\{Y_t\}$ is said to be completely stationary or strict sense stationary (abbreviated as SSS) if the process Y_t and Y_{t+n} have the same statistics for any$n$. So, the characteristics$Y_{(t+n)}$, for all n, will be the same asY_t.

Non-Stationary Processes

A big reason for using a stationary data sequence instead of a non-stationary sequence is that non-stationary sequences, usually, are more complex and take more calculations when forecasting is applied to a data series (Beusekom, 2003).

Where a series submit over time variation in your parameters, so, we have a series non-stationary, which when submitted to differentiation process becomes stationary. If the time series is not stationary, we can often transform it to stationarity with one of the following way:

a) Difference the data, by create the new series

$$Y_t = X_t - X_{t-1}$$

The differenced data will contain one less point than the original data. Although you can difference the data more than once, one difference is usually sufficient.

b) If the data contain a trend, we can fit some type of curve to the data and then model the residuals from that fit.

c) For non-constant variance, taking the logarithm or square root of the series may stabilize the variance. For negative data, you can add a suitable constant to make all the data positive before applying the transformation. This constant can then be subtracted from the model to obtain predicted (i.e., the fitted) values and forecasts for future points.

White noise

In according of Cochrane (2005), The building block for our time series models is the white noise process, which I'll denoteε_t. In the least general case,

$$\varepsilon_t \sim i.d.d.N\left(0,\sigma_{\varepsilon_t}^2\right)$$

Notice three implications of this assumption:

1. $E(\varepsilon_t)=E(\varepsilon_t \mid \varepsilon_{t-1}, \varepsilon_{t-2}...)=E(\varepsilon_t \mid \text{all information at } t-1)=0$

2. $E(\varepsilon_t\varepsilon_{t-i})=\text{cov}(\varepsilon_t\varepsilon_i)=0$

3. $\text{var}(\varepsilon_t)=\text{var}(\varepsilon_t \mid \varepsilon_{t-1}, \varepsilon_{t-2}...)=\text{var}(\varepsilon_t \mid \text{all information at } t-1)=\sigma^2$

The first and second properties are the absence of any serial correlation or predictability. The third property is conditional homoscedasticity or a constant conditional variance. Later, we will generalize the building block process. For example, we may assume property 2 and 3 without normality, in which case the ε_t need not be independent. We may also assume the first property only, in which case ε_t is a martingale difference sequence (Cochrane, 2005).

Summary of time series models:

Autoregressive models - AR(p)

The class of models purely autoregressive is defined by:

$$Y_t=\frac{a_t}{\varphi_p(B)} \tag{15}$$

where $\varphi_p(B)$ has p coefficients. The AR (p) assumes that the result is the weighted sum of its p past values than white noise.

The condition of stationarity of the AR (p) states that all the p roots of the characteristic equation fall outside the unit circle (Russo, et al, 2006).

Moving average models - MA(q)

According to Russo, et al (2009), the class of moving averages models is defined by

$$Y_t=\theta_q(B)a_t \tag{16}$$

where $\theta_q(B)$ has q coefficients. The models MA (q) resulting from the linear combination of random shocks that occurred during the current and past periods.

The invertibility condition requires that all roots of the characteristic equation fall outside the unit circle.

Autoregressive and moving average models - ARMA (p,q)

The class of models, autoregressive-moving average is of type

$$Y_t=\frac{\theta_q(B)a_t}{\varphi_p(B)} \tag{17}$$

where $\varphi_p(B)$has p coefficients and $\theta_q(B)$ has q coefficients. With a combination of models AR (p) and MA (q), it is expected that the models ARMA (p,q) be models extremely parsimonious, using few coefficients to explain the same serie.

From the standpoint of adjustment, it is very important because you can adjust more quickly. The condition of stationary and invertibility of a ARMA (p, q) require that all p roots of f (B) 0 and all the q roots of q (B) 0 fall outside the unit circle (Russo, et al, 2009).

Autoregressive Integrated Moving Averages Models - ARIMA (p,d,q)

The class of autoregressive-integrated-moving-average models are defined by the equation,

$$Y_t = \frac{\theta_q(B)a_t}{\varphi_p(B)(1-B)^d} \tag{18}$$

to an integrator positive *d*. Made the differentiation of the series *d* times necessary to make it stationary, then the ARIMA(p, d, q) model can be adjusted through the ARMA(p,q) model (Russo, et al, 2009).

Sazonal Model - SARIMA

According to Fischer (1982), the appearance of some short-term cyclical behavior is called seasonality. For a full treatment about series of time, need to characterize and eliminate this cyclic function of time to become the condition of stationarity.

Seasonality means a tendency to repeat a certain behavior of the variable that occurs with some regularity in time. That is, are those series that have variations of a similar amount of time to another, characterized by showing high serial correlation between observations of the variable spaced by the period of seasonality, and, of course, the serial correlation between the next observations.

Similar to the process ARIMA (p,d,q) this process develops the model in one of three basic forms of description of each value ofY_t, and applies the same procedures developed for a model where the seasonal component is not present. After establishing the value of the variable in period t+h, then applies the expectancy operator. Forecast errors, confidence intervals and updating are treated similarly to the ARIMA model (Fischer, 1982).

Box-Jenkins Methodology

This method for the prediction is based on the setting called tentative ARIMA models, has a flexible modeling methodology that forecasts are made from the current and past values of these series. Therefore, describing both the stationary behavior as the non-stationary zero. ARIMA models are able to describe the process of generating a variety of series for forecasters (corresponding to the filters) without taking into account the economic relations, for example that generated the series (Morretin and Toloi, 2006).

The determination of the best model for "Box and Jenkins" methodology following this steps (Leroy, 2006):

Identification

Identification is the most critical phase of the "Box and Jenkins" methodology, it is possible that several researchers to identify different models for the same series, using different criteria of choice (ACF, PACF, [illegible]). Typically the models should be parsimonious. The study analyzes the ACF and PACF, and attempts to identify the model. The [illegible] to determine the order of (p,d,q), based on the behavior of the Autocorrelation Functions (ACF) and Partial Autocorrelation (PACF), as well as their respective correlograms.

Estimation:

After identifying the best model should then adjust and examine it. The adjusted models are compared using several criteria. One of the criteria is the of parsimony, in which it appears that the incorporation of coefficients additional improves the degree of adjustment (increases the R^2 and reduces the sum of squared residuals) model, but you reduces the degrees of freedom. One of ways to improve the degree of adjustment of this model to time series data is to include lags additional in Cases AR (p), MA (q), ARMA (p, q) and ARIMA.

The inclusion of additional lags implies increasing the number of repressors, which leads to a reduction in the sum of squared residuals estimated. Currently, there are several criteria for selection of models that generate a trade-off between reductions in the sum of squared residuals and estimated a more parsimonious model.

Generally, when working with lagged variables are lost about the time series under study. Therefore, to compare alternative models (or competitors) should remain fixed number of information used for all models compared.

Checking:

Aspiring to know the efficacy of the model found, takes place waste analysis. If the residuals are autocorrelated, then the dynamics of the series is not completely explained by the coefficients of the fitted model. It should be excluded from the process of choosing the model(s) with this feature.

An analysis of existence (or not) of serial autocorrelation of waste is made based on the functions of autocorrelation and partial autocorrelation of waste and their respective correlograms. It is noteworthy that, when estimating a model, it is desired that the error produced by it have characteristic "white noise" that is, this will be independent and identically distributed (i.i.d. condition).

Forecast:

Predictions can be ex-ante, made to calculate future values of short-term variable in the study. Or, ex-post held to generate values within the sample period. The better these last, the more efficient the model estimated. We choose the best model throught the lower Mean Absolute Percentage Error (MAPE). It is a formal measure of the quality of forecasts ex-post. Therefore, the lower value of the MAPE is the best fit of forecasts of the model to time series data.

5. Methodology and Results

In this work we analyzed the Têxtil Oeste Ltda industry, whose Statistical Control of Processes implantation happened in 1999. Here, we limited to analyze the control charts for continuous variables as tools used for the control of the process. The conventional Shewhart control charts were used added of other appropriated models to transformations of autocorrelations data in data that are independent and usually distributed.

In thread's polypropylene process there are several outputs to consider critical. One of these outputs is the thread's resistance. In an effort to develop a control plan to assure quality of the appropriate surface, it was certain that the resistance has a main impact on surface quality of the thread. So, to verify the quality of the thread, it's resistance should be controlled.

At once, the data used in this study is the daily data of the thread's polypropylene resistances control.

These data are for the models identification and estimation and for the models predictive capacity analysis. Before control charts be applied, three fundamental assumptions must be met: The process is under control; the data are normally distributed; and the observations are independent.

Montgomey (2009) considers that the points out of control are stipulated reasonably well for the controls charts of Shewhart when the normality assumption is somewhat violated, but when observations aren't independent, control charts yield deceiving results. Many processes don't produce independent observations. Alwan (1991) describes a method for control charting with autocorrelated data. The method involves fitting a time series curve and control charting the residuals.

It was made a study that helped to verify where it is the largest instability of the process, so that we can make a better control of the system. It is suspected that the daily thread's resistance data aren't independent, and the result of a plot of these data, as showing in Figure 4, supports this belief.

The problem is to implement statistical control for a process that has autocorrelation (Dobson, 1995). The Figure 4 shows us the great data variability. Calculations were performed to confirm the autocorrelation's suspected.

Calculations were done to confirm the suspected autocorreation. The autocorrelation coefficient for thread's resistance is defined as

$$r_k = \frac{\sum_{t=1}^{n-k} (x_t - \bar{x})(x_{t+k} - \bar{x})}{\sum_{t=1}^{n} (x_t - \bar{x})^2}, \; k = 0,1,2, \; \ldots$$

where k = time periods ahead

n = total number of data

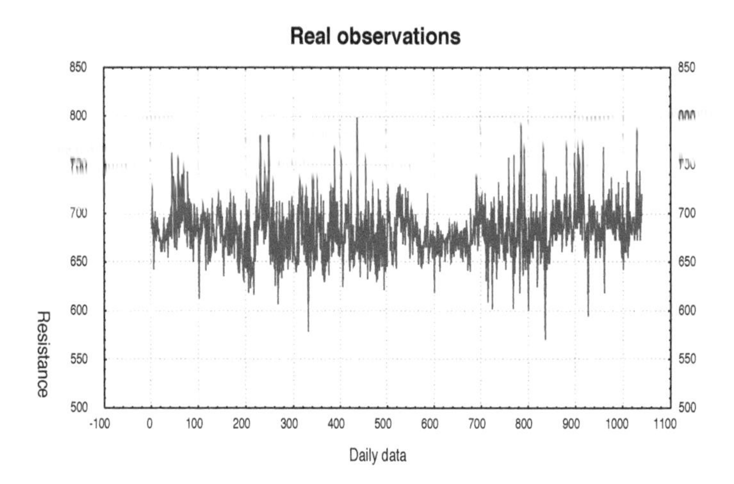

Figure 4. Daily data.

The standard error at lag k, if $k = 1$ is $Se_k = \sqrt{\frac{1}{n}}$, and the standard error at lag k, if $k1$ is

$$Se_k = \sqrt{\frac{1}{n}\left(1 + 2\sum_{i=1}^{k-1} r_i^2\right)}$$

The autocorrelation coefficient for $k = 1$ and $k = 2$are:

$$r_1 = \frac{160680,24}{971034} = 0,16$$

and

$$r_2 = \frac{100113,10}{971034} = 0,10$$

The standard error for $k = 1$ and $k = 2$are:

$$Se_1 = \sqrt{\frac{1}{1041}} = 0,0310$$

and

$$Se_2 = \sqrt{\frac{1}{1041}\left[1 + 2(0,16)^2\right]} = 0,0317$$

The Figure 5 shows the autocorrelation coefficients and 2 standard errors for these coefficients for up to 24 lags, and the Figure 6 shows the partial autocorrelation coefficients and the 2 standard errors for these coefficients for up to 24 lags.

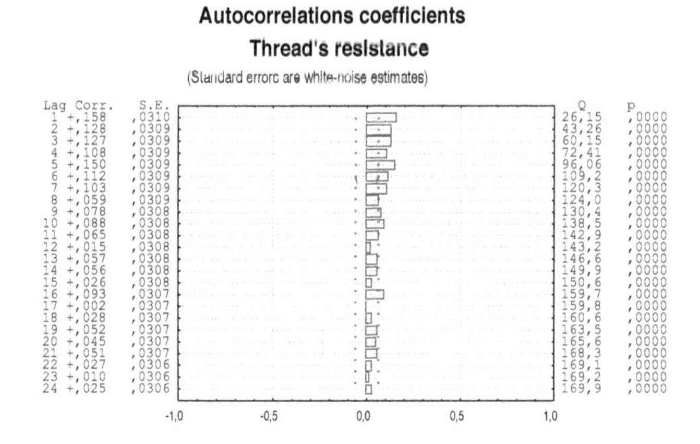

Figure 5. Autocorrelations coefficients.

As we can see, the data are highly autocorrelated. The autocorrelation coefficients for lags 1-7 exceed two the standard errors. Before a control charts can be used, these data must be transformed to guarantee the independence of each observation.

To find an independent, normally distributed data set, Montgomery (2009) recommends to model the structure and to develop the control charting of the residuals directly.

The Box & Jenkins's methodology was used, to determine the parameters of the model (Box, Jenkins and Reinsel, 2008).

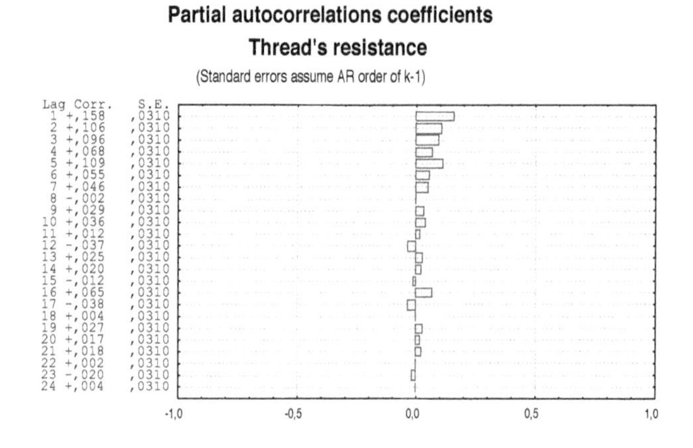

Figure 6. Partial autocorrelations coefficients.

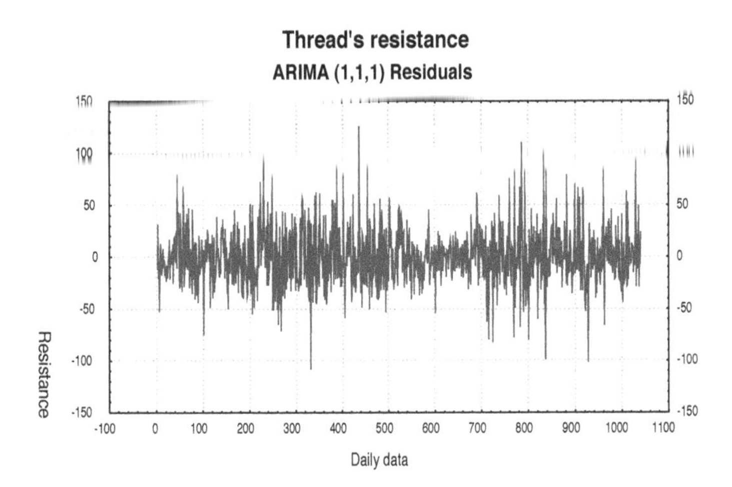

Figure 7. Residuals of thread's resistance.

The Figures 8 and 9 show that the obtained model is adapted to the resistance data. The autocorrelation coefficients were calculated for the transformed data defined for the model ARIMA (1,1,1), to validate that the autocorrelation has been removed from the data.

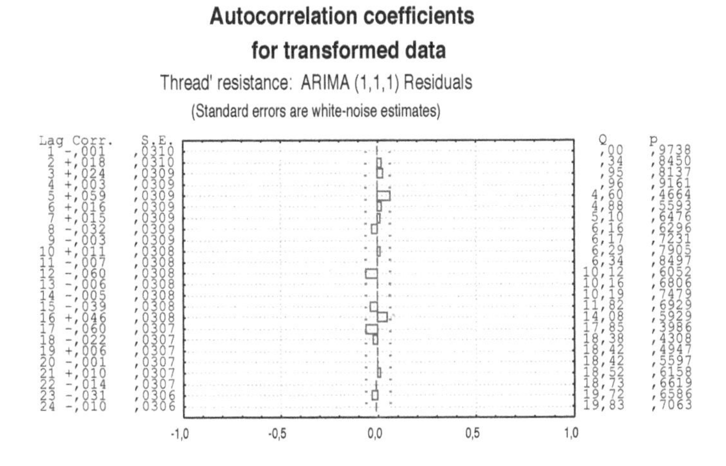

Figure 8. Autocorrelation coefficients.

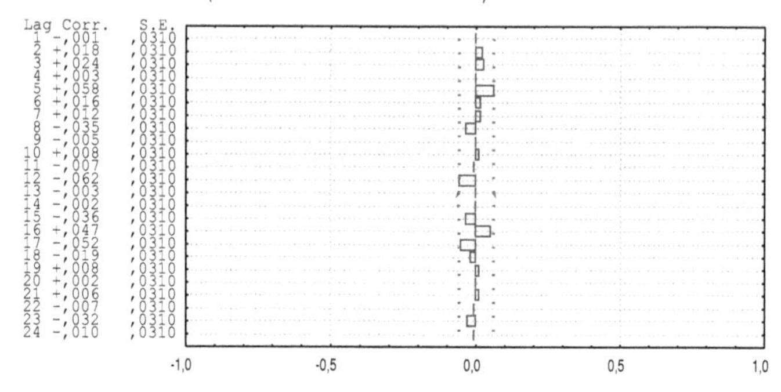

Figure 9. Partial autocorrelations coefficients for transformed data.

Figure 8 and 9 show that the defined data is independent from an observation to another observation. And the table 1 shows the Chi-square test to verify the normality.

For two degrees of freedom, $\chi^2_{0,05}$=5,991. As the calculation qui-square value was χ^2= 5,0415, and it is smaller than the critical value, the data are considered as normal. Now the behavior of the productive process can be verified.

The Chi-square test was executed, to verify the normality:

Lower Limit	Upper Limit	Obs	Exp	$(Obs-Exp)^2$/ Exp
649,0708	743,3123	744	696,1916	3,2831
648,9230	743,4601	672	696,1916	0,8406
648,7757	743,6074	702	696,1916	0,0485
648,6288	743,7543	690	696,1916	0,0551
648,4823	743,9008	720	696,1916	0,8142
Total				5,0415

Table 1. Test the Chi-square.

Figure 10 shows ($\overline{X}$) and (S) charts for the real data.

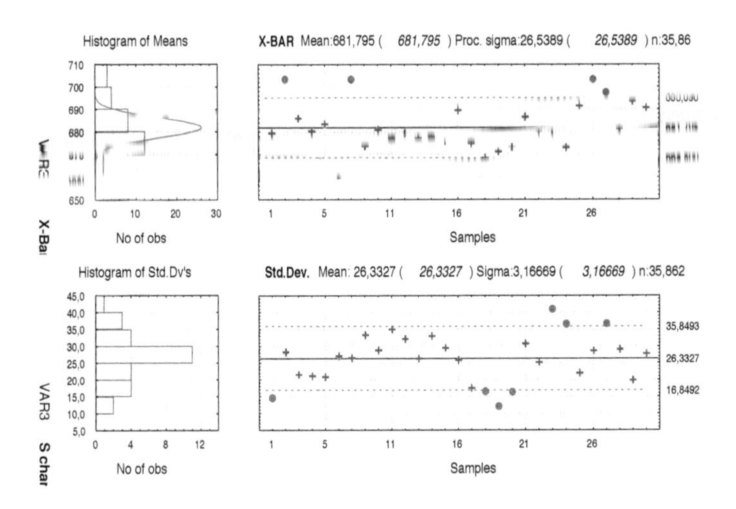

Figure 10. $\bar{X}$ and S charts for real data.

Through the illustration 10 we can notice the sequence of observations and limits of the traditional Shewhart charts, where several points were out of the control limits, indicating that the process is apparently out of control. In fact, before the transformation of the data, we found the data really correlated what took us to model for a process ARIMA (Wardell, Moskowitz and Plante, 1994).

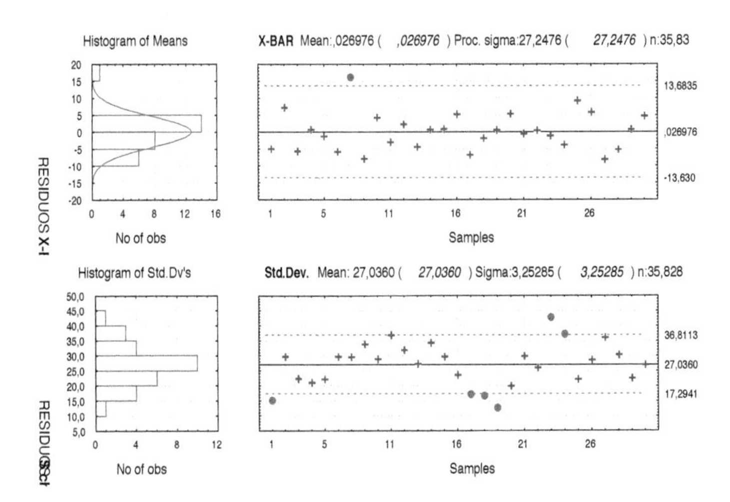

Figure 11. ($\bar{X}$) and (S) charts for transformed data.

Figure 11 shows ($\overline{X}$) and (S) charts for transformed data. Verifications revealed that the system had been drained during this time period and actions were taken to correct the problem. The problem was in the first observations, which were ignored, the normality condition was verified, and the control charts X and S were replotted.

Through the Figure 11 we can observe that the control charts for the same data, indicate that the residual values are practically inside of control limits for the average. According to Wardell, Moskowitz and Plant (1994) it is entirely possible in traditional control charts, the points are out of the limits because of the systematic or the common causes and not because of occurrence of special causes.

6. Conclusion

According to Reid and Sanders (2002), there are several types of statistical quality control (SQC) techniques. One category of SQC techniques consists of descriptive statistics tools such as the mean, range, and standard deviation. These tools are used to describe quality characteristics and relationships. Another category of SQC techniques consists of statistical process control (SPC) methods that are used to monitor changes in the production process. To understand SPC methods you must understand the differences between common and assignable causes of variation.

Common causes of variation are based on random causes that cannot be identified. A certain amount of common or normal variation occurs in every process due to differences in materials, workers, machines, and other factors. Assignable causes of variation, on the other hand, are variations that can be identified and eliminated. An important part of statistical process control (SPC) is monitoring the production process to make sure that the only variations in the process are those due to common or normal causes. Under these conditions we say that a production process is in a state of control. You should also understand the different types of quality control charts that are used to monitor the production process: x-bar charts, R-range charts, p-charts, and c-charts, Reid and Sanders (2002).

In this chapter we show how to use the techniques of quality control for autocorrelated data. Thus, the data collected were analyzed simultaneously, the continuous variables, to find a possible reason for lack of control in the final stages of production. We presented methods for using the techniques of statistical quality control for correlated observations. It is the autocorrelation data, is modeled by the continuous variables ARIMA. With the residuals obtained in the models, we applied the Shewhart control charts.

The traditional Shewhart control charts can be used for process control, even when the assumptions of independent observations are transgressed, by removing the autocorrelation with a time series models. For applying those techniques, the thread's resistance stayed in control state for the average. The result was a decrease in the variation of surface quality of the polypropylene thread that is produced, while simultaneously it increased the surface quality average.

Many companies, because they believe in the advantages that can be obtained from the practice of SQC, invest many resources in the implementation, especially of the conventional control charts, called Shewhart charts. Since it is not necessary to a thorough knowledge of statistics, is more favorable to the deployment of these graphs by the companies, but not always the results are as expected. There is a concern with the correlation of data.

In this context, the text presented throughout this chapter can serve as a reference to the industries that face difficulties in deploying statistical quality control. However, one must be careful with the type of variables to analyze what is being proposed, which allows us to conclude that this proposed combination of techniques for time series with control charts, claim to be complete and extended to cover all possible difficulties we can find. In the classic model of monitoring, there is no such information to identify an non conform item, in the end of teh proces, no one knows how to do for the same does not happen, because the variables used in the previous process are autocorrelated.

Author details

Suzana Leitão Russo[1*], Maria Emilia Camargo[2] and Jonas Pedro Fabris[3]

*Address all correspondence to: suzana.ufs@hotmail.com

1 Department of Statistic - Federal University of Sergipe, Brazil

2 Post-Graduate Program in Administration, University of Caxias of South, Brazil

3 Fabris Industry, Brazil

References

[1] Alwan, L. C. (1991). Autocorrelation: fixed versus variable control limits quality and reliability. *Engineering International*, 4(2), 167-188.

[2] Beusekom, D. P. V. (2003). Forecasting & Detrending Of Time Series Models. University of Amsterdam. Faculty of Sciences Study Bedrijfswiskunde & Informatica. (www.few.vu.nl/.../werkstuk-beusekom_tcm39-91323.html acess in Apr, 05, 2012).

[3] Box, G. E. P., Jenkins, G. M., & Reinsel, G. C. (2008). Series Analysis: Forecasting and Control. Wiley Series in Probability and Statistics: 4 Ed.

[4] Chen, A., & Elsayed, E. A. (2000). An alternative mean estimator for processes monitored by SPC charts. *Int. J. Prod. Res.*, 38(13), 3093-3109.

[5] Camargo, M. E., & Russo, S. L. (2011). Modeling and forecasting tourist traffic in the Mauá and Alba Posse Harbors. *African Journal of Business Management*, 5(2), 433-439, 18 January.

[6] Cochrane, J. H. (2005). Time Series for Macroeconomics and Finance. Chicago: Spring.

[7] Dobson, B. (1995). Control charting dependent data: a case study. *Quality Engineering*, 7(4), 757-768.

[8] Jiang, W., Tsui, K., & Woodall, W. (2000). A new SPC monitoring method: the ARMA chart. *Technometrics*, 399-410.

[9] Fischer, S. (1982). Séries Univariantes de Tempo-Metodologia Box and Jenkins. Porto Alegre- RS, Fundação de Economia e Estatística.

[10] Juran, J. M. (1993). Made in U.S.A.: A renaissance in quality. *Harvard Business Review*, July-August, 42-50.

[11] Loureço Filho, R. C. B. (1964). Controle Estatístico de Qualidade. Rio de Janeiro: Livro Tec. S/A.

[12] Montgomery, D. C. (2009). Introduction to Statistical Quality Control. Vol. 1, 6 Ed., USA: John Wiley & Sons.

[13] Morettin, P. A., & Toloi, C. M. (2006). Análise de Séries Temporais. Ed Edgard Blucher. São Paulo.

[14] Panagiotidou, S. (2009). An economically designed, integrated quality and maintenance model using an adaptive Shewhart chart. *Reliability Engineering & System Safety*, 94(3), 732-741.

[15] Reid, R. D., & Sanders, N. R. (2002). Operations Management. 3rd Edition. John Willey & Sons.

[16] Russo, S., Rodrigues, P. M. M., & Camargo, M. E. (2006). Aplicação de Séries Temporais na Série Teor de Umidade da Areia de Fundição da Indústria Fundimisa. *Revista Gestão Industrial*, 1808-0448, 2(1), 35-45, Universidade Tecnológica Federal do Paraná-UTFPR, Campus Ponta Grossa- Paraná- Brasil, D.O.I.: 10.3895/S1808-04482006000100004.

[17] Shewhart, W. A. (1931). Economic control of quality of the manufactured product. Van Nostrand, New York.

[18] Wardell, D. G., Moskowitz, H., & Plante, R. (1994). Run-length distribuitions of special-cause control charts for correlates process. *Technometrics*, 36(1), 3-16.

[19] Werkema, M. C. C. (1995). Ferramentas Estatísticas Básicas para o Gerenciamento de Processos. Belo Horizonte: Ed. Líttera Maciel Ltda, Vol II.

Section 2

Total Quality Management

Chapter 4

Formation of Product Properties Determining Its Quality in a Multi-Operation Technological Process

Andrey Rostovtsev

Additional information is available at the end of the chapter

1. Introduction

Quality management of manufacture products requires knowledge of the values and interaction of all factors which form the quality. The mathematical description or the model of the process for obtaining the required product properties which correspond to the specified quality are needed for this purpose in the first place.

One of the most widespread processes in machine-building manufacture is the multi-operation technological process. As known, formation of product properties starts from receiving blank parts or raw materials to the enterprise warehouse for subsequent processing or reprocessing. After blanking operations, the main technological operations (TOs) are performed, which in most cases are concluded by final assembling. Sometimes final surface finishing and/or deposition of coating is performed after assembling.

During formation of product properties it is necessary to take into account the measurement errors which inevitably appear during quality control at each TO. In general, the technological process may be considered as a set of successive technologic states (TS) E[1)][1], in which the property index (PI) or a set of PIs obtained at the completed TO have passed quality control and keep their values unchanged. This allows representing the technological process in the form of a tuple

$$E_1 \prec E_2 \prec \ldots \prec E_r \prec \ldots \prec E_{s-1} \prec E_s, \; r = \overline{1,s} \tag{1}$$

where:

$\prec$ is the symbol of ordered preference in the sense of closeness to the final TS;

r and s are the subscripts of current TS and final TS, respectively.

The question now arises: what should be regarded as parallel transformation of the properties considered here? Undoubtedly, assembling TOs should. Here this tuple is expressed in another form:

$$(E_1, E_2, ..., E_r, ..., E_{s-1})^T \prec E_s, \quad (2)$$

where T is the sign of transposition of several E_r in vectorial form of recording.[1]

In case of such, so to say, 'existential' approach to formation of product properties, TS E_r must be considered as achieving of the prescribed value by property P_r at the completed TO or, in vectorial form, as achieving of the prescribed values by a set of properties (P_r), which is testified by the PIs obtained as the result of post-operation check.

For the development of mathematical model of formation of product properties (expressed by relevant PIs) during technological process, it is essential to represent each TO in the form of elementary oriented graph (fig.1), which nodes correspond to adjacent TSs (preceding TS E_{r-1} and subsequent TS E_r), respectively [1]. Graph edge r oriented at TS E_r is symbolizing a TO or, if it is principally significant, a technological step, during which the property P_r or properties (P_r) are transformed from TS E_{r-1} into TS E_r, as shown in fig. 1 a and 1b, respectively.

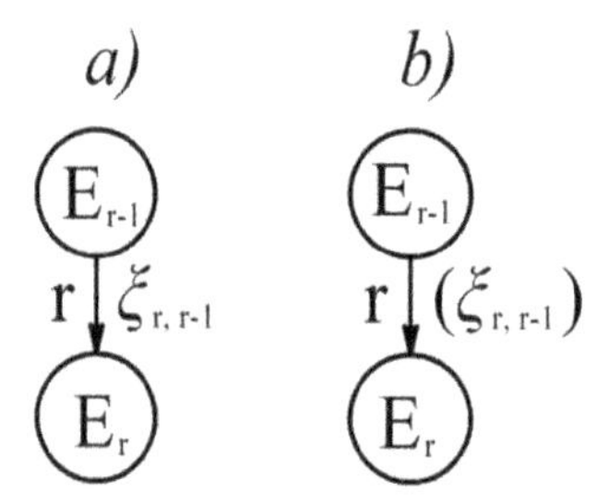

Figure 1. Mathematical model of a technological operation r of transformation of one (a) or several (b) property indices of a product from technological state E_{r-1} into technological state E_r with transformation coefficients ξr,r-1 or (ξr,r-1), respectively.

For each PI achieved by TS E_r, it is convenient to split the combined random error $\omega^2_{r_\Sigma}$ into three components: inherent error ω_r, extrinsic error ψ_r (carried from the previous TO or TOs), and check error κ_r, with the following equation valid for the variances of these errors [2–4]:

$$\omega^2_{r_\Sigma} = \omega^2_r + \psi^2_r + \kappa^2_r. \quad (3)$$

1 Initial letter of the word «Existence» – state (French)

Neglecting the infinitely small quantities of higher orders, formula (3) allows transition to the product properties transformation coefficient

$$\xi_{r,r-1_\Sigma} = \psi_r / \omega_{r-1_\Sigma} \tag{4}$$

However, it should be noted that in some cases, where functional connection between coefficient $\xi_{r,r-1}$ and PI exists in some or other form, it is not possible to neglect these infinitely small quantities of higher orders[2]. This coefficient is considered here as "weight" of edge r, fig. 1.

In case of several PIs, formulas (3) and (4) may be written in vectorial-matrix form:

$$(\omega_{r_\Sigma}^2) = (\omega_r^2) + (\psi_r^2) + (\kappa_r^2), \tag{5}$$

where round brackets denote vectorial form of the relevant errors, and

$$(\xi_{r,r-1_\Sigma}) = (\psi_r) / (\omega_{r-1_\Sigma}), \tag{6}$$

where $(\xi_{r,r-1_\Sigma})$ is the matrix of transformation of PI from TS r-1 to TS r.

Passing to the nonrandom component Δ_{r_Σ} of PI combined error, it is necessary to tie its center of grouping to zero reference point which corresponds to PI nominal value. Depending on accepted normalization method, such point may be either the middle of PI tolerance zone, or one of the limits (left or right) of PI tolerance zone. These limits represent the so-called functional (if related to E_s) thresholds or technological (in this case) thresholds [4–6], left $x_{\ulcorner}$ and right $x_{\urcorner}$.

Hence, the requirements to PI may be represented for each of these thresholds by semi-open intervals

$$x \geq x_{\ulcorner},\ [x_{\ulcorner}, \infty) \text{ and } x \leq x_{\urcorner}, (0, x_{\urcorner}], \tag{7}$$

respectively, and for the tolerance zone – by segment

$$x_{\ulcorner} \leq x \leq x_{\urcorner}, [x_{\ulcorner}, x_{\urcorner}], \tag{8}$$

allowing to place PI values on x number axis.

2 E.g., in case of assembling fuel-regulating components of gas turbine engines.

If TS E_r contains several non-random combined errors (Δ_{r_Σ}), they may be united, similar to random errors, into the common vector of displacement of their centers of grouping. Therefore, the non-random analog of formula (5) will be:

$$(\Delta_{r_\Sigma}) = (\Delta\omega_r) + (\Delta\psi_r) + (\Delta\kappa_r), \tag{9}$$

where $\Delta\kappa r$ is set to zero because of assumed centrality of measurement errors distribution (systematic error of measurements must be close to zero due to timely certification and calibration of measuring instruments).

Then formula (9) will take the form

$$(\Delta_{r_\Sigma}) = (\Delta\omega_r) + (\Delta\psi_r), \tag{10}$$

Then it is necessary to reveal the inversion of PI errors, showing how the errors from the previous TSs migrate to subsequent TSs, and to perform, so to say, their mathematical convolution, uniting them into appropriate mathematical expressions [2–4, 6]. Let us start from consecutive transformation of errors of random PI components.

Thus, as mentioned earlier, blank parts or raw materials are received to the enterprise warehouse. Naturally, their PI has a combined error ω_{1_Σ} specified by delivery terms (at first, let us consider the simplest case of inversion of a single PI). In this case inversion starts from TS E_1 with combined technological error ω_{1_Σ}, and its first step is: transition from TS E_1 to TS E_2, with quadratic transformation of error variances corresponding to this step

$$\omega_{2_\Sigma}^2 = \omega_2^2 + \psi_2^2 + \kappa_2^2 = \omega_2^2 + \xi_{21}^2\omega_{1_\Sigma}^2 + \kappa_2^2. \tag{11}$$

The second step performs transition from TS E_2 to TS E_3, which is characterized by two quadratic transformations:

$$\begin{aligned} \omega_{3_\Sigma}^2 &= \omega_3^2 + \psi_3^2 + \kappa_3^2 = \omega_3^2 + \xi_{32}^2\omega_{2_\Sigma}^2 + \kappa_3^2 = \\ &= \omega_3^2 + \xi_{32}^2(\omega_2^2 + \xi_{21}^2\omega_{1_\Sigma}^2 + \kappa_2^2) + \kappa_3^2 = \\ &= \omega_3^2 + \xi_{32}^2\omega_2^2 + \xi_{32}^2\xi_{21}^2\omega_{1_\Sigma}^2 + \xi_{32}^2\kappa_2^2 + \kappa_3^2. \end{aligned} \tag{12}$$

Structure of formula (12) contains the forming, so to say, nucleus of inversion of manufacturing errors, or the inversion nucleus:

$$\xi_{32}^2\omega_2^2 + \xi_{32}^2\xi_{21}^2\omega_{1_\Sigma}^2 \tag{13}$$

Using the method of mathematical induction, let us try to find out the tendencies of subsequent evolution of this nucleus in course of approaching to the final TS. For this purpose, let us perform similar quadratic transformations on the third step of inversion

$$\omega_{4_\Sigma}^2 = \omega_4^2 + \psi_4^2 + \kappa_4^2 = \omega_4^2 + \xi_{43}^2\omega_{3_\Sigma}^2 + \kappa_4^2 = \omega_4^2 + \xi_{43}^2(\omega_3^2 + \xi_{32}^2\omega_2^2 + \xi_{32}^2\xi_{21}^2\omega_{1_\Sigma}^2 + \xi_{32}^2\kappa_2^2 + \kappa_3^2) + \kappa_4^2 = \omega_4^2 + \xi_{43}^2\omega_3^2 + \xi_{43}^2\xi_{32}^2\omega_2^2 + \xi_{43}^2\xi_{32}^2\xi_{21}^2\omega_{1_\Sigma}^2 + \xi_{43}^2\xi_{32}^2\kappa_2^2 + \xi_{43}^2\kappa_3^2) + \kappa_4^2. \tag{14}$$

and on the fourth step of inversion

$$\omega_{5_\Sigma}^2 = \omega_5^2 + \psi_5^2 + \kappa_5^2 = \omega_5^2 + \xi_{54}^2\omega_{4_\Sigma}^2 + \kappa_5^2 = \omega_5^2 + \xi_{54}^2(\omega_4^2 + \xi_{43}^2\omega_3^2 + \xi_{43}^2\xi_{32}^2\omega_2^2 + \xi_{43}^2\xi_{32}^2\xi_{21}^2\omega_{1_\Sigma}^2 + \xi_{43}^2\xi_{32}^2\kappa_2^2 + \xi_{43}^2\kappa_3^2 + \kappa_4^2) + \kappa_5^2 = \omega_5^2 + \xi_{54}^2\omega_4^2 + \xi_{54}^2\xi_{43}^2\omega_3^2 + \xi_{54}^2\xi_{43}^2\xi_{32}^2\omega_2^2 + \xi_{54}^2\xi_{43}^2\xi_{32}^2\xi_{21}^2\omega_{1_\Sigma}^2 + \xi_{54}^2\xi_{43}^2\xi_{32}^2\kappa_2^2 + \xi_{54}^2\xi_{43}^2\kappa_3^2 + \xi_{54}^2\kappa_4^2 + \kappa_5^2. \tag{15}$$

Formula (14) shows quite evidently the general tendencies of increase of inversion nucleus components and increase of the inversion structure as a whole. This allows making the first steps for generalization and more convenient perception of the results obtained.

To improve visual appearance of formula (14), let us introduce the generalizing coefficient Ξ_{s1}, denoting it as multiplicative coefficient of PI transformation. For s-1 linear transformations of PI, this coefficient is the product:

$$\Xi_{s1} = \xi_{21}\xi_{32}...\xi_{r,r-1}...\xi_{s,s-1} = \prod_{r=2}^{s}\xi_{r,r-1}. \tag{16}$$

Similarly, for quadratic transformation of errors characterized by $\xi_{r,r-1}^2$:

$$\Xi_{s1}^2 = \xi_{21}^2\xi_{32}^2...\xi_{r,r-1}^2...\xi_{s,s-1}^2 = \prod_{r=2}^{s}\xi_{r,r-1}^2. \tag{17}$$

Now formula (14) may be rewritten in a simpler manner:

$$\omega_{5\Sigma}^2 = \omega_5^2 + \xi_{54}^2\omega_4^2 + \Xi_{53}^2\omega_3^2 + \Xi_{52}^2\omega_2^2 + \Xi_{51}^2\omega_{1_\Sigma}^2 + \Xi_{52}^2\kappa_2^2 + \Xi_{53}^2\kappa_3^2 + \Xi_{54}^2\kappa_4^2 + \kappa_5^2. \tag{18}$$

Then let us generalize formula (17) for arbitrary number s of TSs, with parallel combining of similar terms:

$$\begin{aligned}\omega_{s_\Sigma}^2 &= \omega_s^2 + \Xi_{s,s\text{-}1}^2(\omega_{s\text{-}1}^2 + \kappa_{s\text{-}1}^2) + \Xi_{s,s\text{-}2}^2(\omega_{s\text{-}2}^2 + \kappa_{s\text{-}2}^2) + \ldots + \\ &+ \Xi_{s,r}^2(\omega_r^2 + \kappa_r^2) + \ldots \Xi_{s,2}^2(\omega_2^2 + \kappa_2^2) + \Xi_{s,1_\Sigma}^2 \omega_{1_\Sigma}^2 + \kappa_s^2.\end{aligned} \tag{19}$$

The following step for generalization of the results obtained will be introduction in formula (18) of the operator $\sum\limits_{r=3}^{s}$ for summing multiplicative coefficients $\Xi_{r,r\text{-}1}$ of transformation for the current index r which is the number of TSs, i.e. $\sum\limits_{r=3}^{s} \Xi_{r,r\text{-}1}^2$:

$$\omega_{s_\Sigma}^2 = \omega_s^2 + \sum_{r=3}^{s} \Xi_{r,r\text{-}1}^2(\omega_{r\text{-}1}^2 + \kappa_{r\text{-}1}^2) + \Xi_{s,1}^2 \omega_{1_\Sigma}^2 + \kappa_s^2, \tag{20}$$

representing the mathematical convolution of combined limiting error ω_{s_Σ} in the technological process containing s TOs performed consecutively.

In case of parallel execution of TOs, as mentioned above, the mathematical convolution on the basis of formula (2) will be

$$\omega_{s_\Sigma}^2 = \xi_{s,1_\Sigma}^2 \omega_{1_\Sigma}^2 + \xi_{s,2_\Sigma}^2 \omega_{2_\Sigma}^2 + \ldots + \xi_{s,r_\Sigma}^2 \omega_{r_\Sigma}^2 + \ldots + \xi_{s,s\text{-}1_\Sigma}^2 \omega_{s\text{-}1_\Sigma}^2 \tag{21}$$

or in concise form

$$\omega_{s_\Sigma}^2 = \sum_{r=1}^{s\text{-}1} \xi_{s,r}^2 \omega_{r_\Sigma}^2 \tag{22}$$

Now it is possible to consider in detail the structure of formulas (19) and (20). Formula (19) contains two inversion nuclei: the main nucleus

$$\sum_{r=3}^{s} \Xi_{r,r\text{-}1}^2(\omega_{r\text{-}1}^2 + \kappa_{r\text{-}1}^2) \tag{23}$$

and additional nucleus

$$\Xi_{s1}^2(\omega_{1_\Sigma}^2) \tag{24}$$

The additional inversion nucleus shows that the error of blank part PI or raw material PI at TS F_1 directly affects PI of the resulting TO F_S regardless of [illegible]. [illegible] again thus demonstrates that special diligence is required for checking incoming blank parts, materials and supplies received from exterior enterprises for reprocessing. Both nuclei are circumposed by intrinsic errors $\omega_S{}^2$ and $\kappa_S{}^2$ of the final, S-th TO; these errors also deserve close attention.

It should be noted that the extrinsic (introduced) error $\psi_{r,}$ is not present in formulas (19) and (20). It may be compared to a sewing needle which does not remain in the fabric sewn by it. As for the parallel transformation of PI errors given by formula (20) is concerned, the inversion of PI errors is performed here in the manner formally identical for all and every TS.

The resulting formula for the non-random component of PI error and consequently performed TOs will look like the linear analog of formula (19):

$$\Delta_{s_\Sigma} = \Delta_s + \sum_{r=3}^{s} \Xi_{r,r\text{-}1}\Delta_{r\text{-}1} + \Xi_{s,1_\Sigma}\Delta_{1_\Sigma} \tag{25}$$

and for TOs performed in parallel – like the linear analog of formula (20):

$$\Delta_{s_\Sigma} = \sum_{r=1}^{s\text{-}1} \xi_{s_\Sigma,r}\Delta_r. \tag{26}$$

For several PIs, according to formulas (5) and

(6), expressions (19) and (20) will become vectorial-matrix expressions, i.e.

$$(\omega^2{}_{s_\Sigma}) = (\omega_s^2) + \sum_{r=3}^{s} (\Xi_{r,r\text{-}1}^2)\left[(\omega_{r\text{-}1}^2) + (\kappa_{r\text{-}1}^2)\right] + (\Xi_{s1}^2)(\omega_{1_\Sigma}^2) + (\kappa_s^2), \tag{27}$$

and

$$(\omega^2{}_{s_\Sigma}) = \sum_{r=1}^{s\text{-}1}\left(\xi_{s,r_\Sigma}^2\right)(\omega_{r_\Sigma}^2), \tag{28}$$

respectively.

The same relates to expressions (21) and (22):

$$(\Delta_{s_\Sigma}) = (\Delta_s) + \sum_{r=3}^{s} (\Xi_{r,r-1})(\Delta_{r-1}) + (\Xi_{s,1})(\Delta_{1_\Sigma}) \tag{29}$$

and

$$(\Delta_{s_\Sigma}) = \sum_{r=1}^{s-1} (\xi_{s_\Sigma,r})(\Delta_r). \tag{30}$$

In formulas (23) – (26), the round brackets indicate vectorial nature of the relevant component, excluding multiplicative transformation coefficients (Ξ_{s1}). These coefficients here are the product of matrices, either linear matrices

$$(\Xi_{s1}) = (\xi_{21})(\xi_{32})...(\xi_{r,r-1})...(\xi_{s-1}) = \prod_{r=2}^{s} (\xi_{r,r-1}) \tag{31}$$

or quadratic matrices

$$(\Xi_{s1}^2) = (\xi_{21}^2)(\xi_{32}^2)...(\xi_{r,r-1}^2)...(\xi_{s,s-1}^2) = \prod_{r=2}^{s} (\xi_{r,r-1}^2) \tag{32}$$

If we consider the consequently performed TOs, then the combined measurement error κ_{s_Σ} accumulated for one PI during the entire technological process in the resultant TS E_S may be obtained from formula (19) in the form

$$(\kappa_{s_\Sigma}^2) = (\kappa_s^2) + \sum_{r=3}^{s} (\Xi_{r,r-1}^2)(\kappa_{r-1}^2) \tag{33}$$

In case of TOs performed in parallel, this error may be expressed according to formula (20) as:

$$(\kappa_{s_\Sigma}^2) = \sum_{r=1}^{s-1} (\xi_{sr_\Sigma}^2)(\kappa_{r_\Sigma}^2). \tag{34}$$

When several PIs are checked, the formulas (29) and (30) will take vectorial-matrix form, i.e.

$$(\kappa_{s_\Sigma}^2) = (\kappa_s^2) + \sum_{r=3}^{s} (\Xi_{r,r-1}^2)(\kappa_{r-1}^2) \tag{35}$$

and

$$(\kappa^2_{s_\Sigma}) = \sum_{r=1}^{s-1} (\zeta^2_{s_r})(\kappa^2_{r_\Sigma}) \quad (36)$$

Formulas (29) – (32) allow determining the share of measurement errors $\kappa^2_{s_\Sigma}$ in the combined error $\omega^2_{s_\Sigma}$ for a single PI as well as for several PIs, $(\kappa^2_{s_\Sigma})$ in $(\omega^2_{s_\Sigma})$, respectively, i.e. $\kappa_{s_\Sigma}/\omega_{s_\Sigma}$ in the resulting TS E_s [6]. For the current, intermediate TSs E_r this relation will have a similar form $\kappa_{r_\Sigma}/\omega_{r_\Sigma}$.

The described above method of mathematical convolution of errors, including measurement errors, in a multi-operational technological process has been applied to production of aggregates for shipbuilding and aerospace industry [3,4,7]. It allows not only revealing, performing mathematical convolution and determining the relationship between PI errors and measurement errors, but also creates prerequisites for comprehensive optimization of measurement errors and selection of measuring instruments at all TOs of a technological process [5].

In connection with broadening introduction of mathematically fuzzy (MF) methods in technological practice [8], it is interesting to know, at least as a first approximation, how the described above may be interpreted in MF form. In the aspect under consideration it is quite often caused by complexity or practical impossibility of actual determination of the value $\xi_{r,r-1}$ or values $(\xi_{r,r-1})$ for transformation coefficients of product PIs using analytical or, so to say, mathematically unfuzzy (MUF) methods. First of all, we are interested in MUF results of forming product PIs in a multi-operational technological process represented by formulas (21 – 26) obtained above.

Let us regard fig. 4, which is a MF analog of fig. 1 for MUF transformation, as the first step in solving this problem. As before, TO here is represented by the oriented graph of transforming PI from TS E_{r-1} into E_r, which edge now symbolizes MF coefficient $\xi_{r/r-1}$ of this transformation.

Formally this coefficient may be supposed to exist as a MF analog of formula (4) – the ratio of dividing two MF numbers in the symbolic notation

$$\boldsymbol{\xi}_{r,r-1} = \boldsymbol{\psi}_r / \boldsymbol{\nu}_{r_{\Sigma-1}}, \quad (37)$$

where $\xi_{r/r-1}$, ψ_r and $\nu_{r_{\Sigma-1}}$ are the components of formula (4) expressed in MF form, highlighted hereinafter by bold type to distinguish from MUF form.

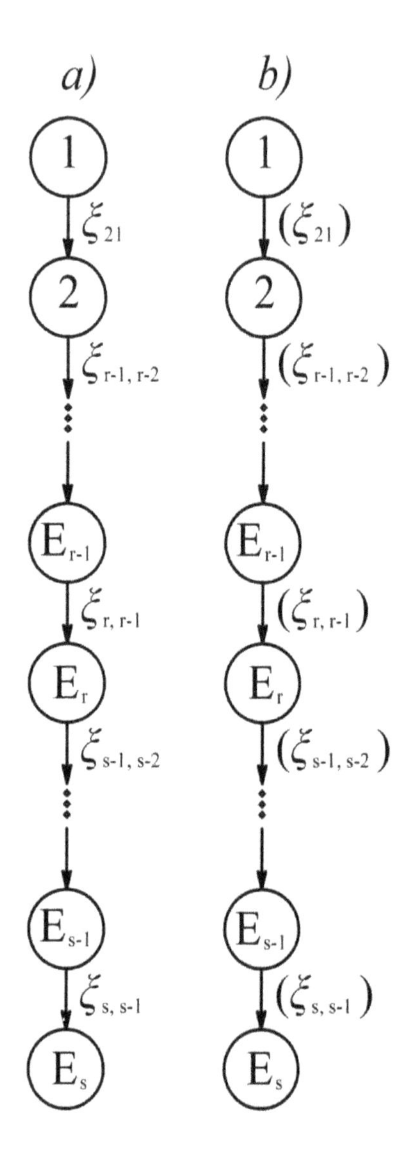

Figure 2. Mathematical model of a technological process with sequential transformation of one (a) or several (b) property indices from the first technological state E_1 into resulting technological state Es with ig

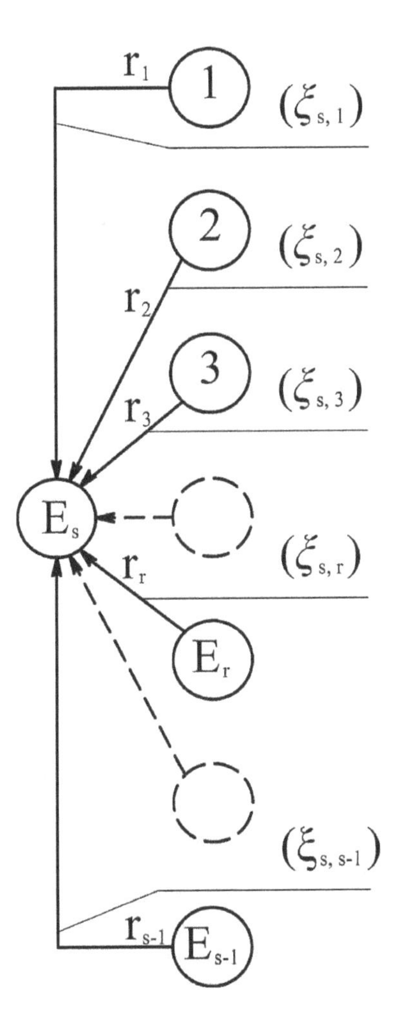

Figure 3. Mathematical model of a technological process with parallel transformation of several property indices from S-1 preceding technological states into one resulting technological state ES by performing r-1 technological operations with transformation coefficients (ξr,r-1).

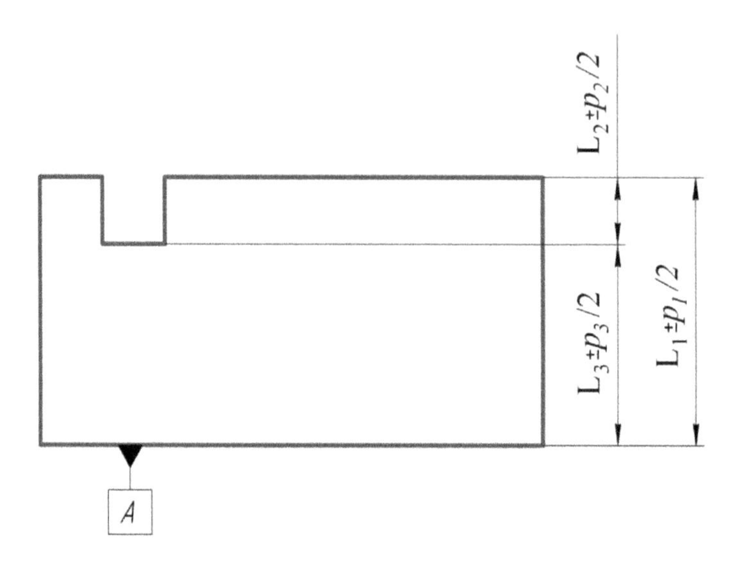

Figure 4. The outline of a component to be measured. ρ_2 – total limiting technologic spread of L_2 dimension, obtained in the process of elaboration of the component production technology,$\rho_{1,\ 3}$ – desired total limiting technologic spreads of L_1 and L_3 dimensions, required for the selection of an appropriate measuring tool.

However, here this ratio in general case is not applicable in the form of transformation coefficient, because MF operations of multiplying and dividing of MF numbers are not inverse to each other. This means that if X and Y are MN numbers, then $X \bullet Y / X \neq Y$. Regrettably, this also holds for operations of algebraic addition and deduction: $(X+Y) - Y \neq X$.

Therefore, in MF case, MUF coefficient $\xi_{r,r\text{-}1}$ may be applied for its direct purpose only in the special case when determined relation exists between MF PIs of adjacent TSs E_r and $E_{r\text{-}1}$. The MF PIs obtained by some or other method shall be brought to mathematical unfuzziness (mathematically cleared)[1)] or defuzzied.

Then the following relationships will be true:

$$\bar{\xi}_{r,r\text{-}1} = \mathrm{B}\psi_r \,/\, \mathrm{B}\nu_{r_{\Sigma\text{-}1}} = \bar{\psi}_r / \bar{\nu}_{r_{\Sigma\text{-}1}}, \tag{38}$$

where:

$B\psi_r$ and $Bv_{r_{\Sigma-1}}$ are carriers (or bases) of MF numbers ψ_r and $v_{r_{\Sigma-1}}$,

$\bar{\psi}_r$ and $\bar{v}_{r_{\Sigma-1}}$ are mathematically cleared (defuzzied) values of MF errors ψ_r and $v_{\Sigma_{r-1}}$, respectively,

« ‾ » is the superscript of mathematical clearing of MF numbers.

It may be noted that $B\psi_r$ and $Bv_{r_{\Sigma-1}}$ are analogs of ψ_r and $v_{\Sigma_{r-1}}$, while $\bar{\psi}_r$ and $\bar{v}_{r_{\Sigma-1}}$ are analogs of $\Delta\psi_r$ and $\Delta v_{r_{\Sigma-1}}$, respectively. This means that both MF data and MUF data are combined in one and the same MF number, allowing to present MF convolution for PI formation by one expression, rather than by two expressions, as in MUF case and in this transitional case.

For this purpose we will have to refer to MF binary relations on classical sets. The latter are a special case of MF sets defined on Cartesian product [9]. In the case under consideration, as shown in [10], for PI of TS E_{r-1} and E_r, there is a fuzzy binary relation of R –order of P_{r-1} and P_r, respectively[3]:

$$P_{r-1} R P_r, \tag{39}$$

which is a fuzzy set with membership function on unfuzzy Cartesian product of two universals P_{r-1} and P_r..

Now let us determine appearance of PI quality check by measurement in MF case. For a single PI x it consists of the following [10]:

- actual value of PI x is determined;
- using inequalities (7) or (8), it is compared with PI value(s) specified in the act on production delivery and acceptance, i. e. with PI functional thresholds $x_{\ulcorner}$ and $x_{\urcorner}$;
- basing on these inequalities, either presence or absence of the relevant property P_x with the product is revealed;
- if property Px is present, the product quality is considered as complying with the requirement imposed on it;
- if property Px is absent, the product quality is considered as non-complying with the requirement imposed on it

In this connection, when MF approach is used, measurement errors on the left $x_{\ulcorner}$ and right $x_{\urcorner}$ functional thresholds and the influence of these errors on the results of product quality control are of interest.

The measurement errors here have the form of the so-called function of membership (FM)

3 "And I saw mathematically clear…" (N.V.Gogol)

$$\eta_x(\theta) = \langle \eta_1 + \eta_2 + \ldots + \eta_\theta + \ldots \eta_\Theta \rangle, \tag{40}$$

where x means the PI measured, ___

θ means current (sequential) number of the term ($\theta = 1,\Theta$),

Θ means overall number of terms,

η means grade of membership (GM) of the term in respect of the measurement result ($0 \le \eta \le 1$),

+ means summation sign, considered as logical only inside angle brackets "< " and " >".

A priori, when knowledge base (in the form of expert estimates, experimental data or some other precedents) is not available, it is reasonable to use the probabilistic FM composed basing on Gaussian normal differential distribution law normalized in regard of mean square deviations. For this purpose, MF unitary normalization of probabilities of this law is additionally used by means of dividing these probabilities by modal value. This value here is assumed equaling to 0.3989. Then these, now Gaussian, FM will look as follows for different Θ:

$$\Theta = 3 \quad \langle 0{,}0110_{-3{,}0\sigma} + 1{,}0000 + 0{,}0110^{+3{,}0\sigma} \rangle, \tag{41}$$

$$\Theta = 5 \quad \langle 0{,}0110_{-3{,}0\sigma} + 0{,}3246_{-1{,}5\sigma} + 1{,}0000 + +0{,}3246^{+1{,}5\sigma} + 0{,}0110^{+3{,}0\sigma} \rangle, \tag{42}$$

$$\Theta = 7 \quad \langle 0{,}0110_{-3{,}0\sigma} + 0{,}1354_{-2{,}0\sigma} + 0{,}6067_{-1{,}0\sigma} + 1{,}0000 + 0{,}6067^{+1{,}0\sigma} + 0{,}1354^{+2{,}0\sigma} + 0{,}0110^{+3{,}0\sigma} \rangle. \tag{43}$$

FM (38) and (39) in graphic form are shown in fig.6 and 7, respectively.

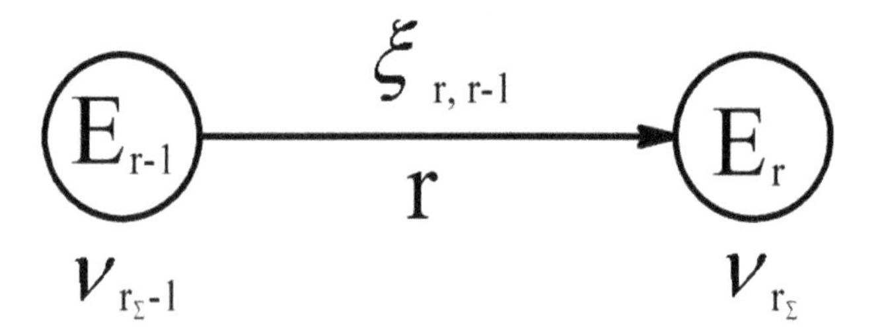

Figure 5. Mathematically fuzzy model of a technological operation r of transformation of one of property indices of a product from technological state E_{r-1} into technological state E_r. v_{r_Σ} and $v_{r_{\Sigma-1}}$ – functions of appurtenance of property indices in the technological states of E_r and E_{r-1}.

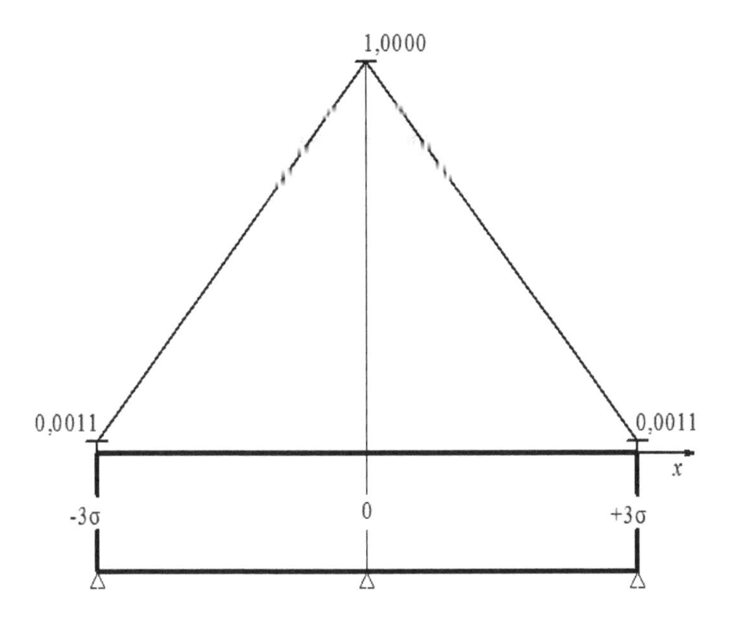

Figure 6. Three-term Gaussian function of membership (Θ = 3).

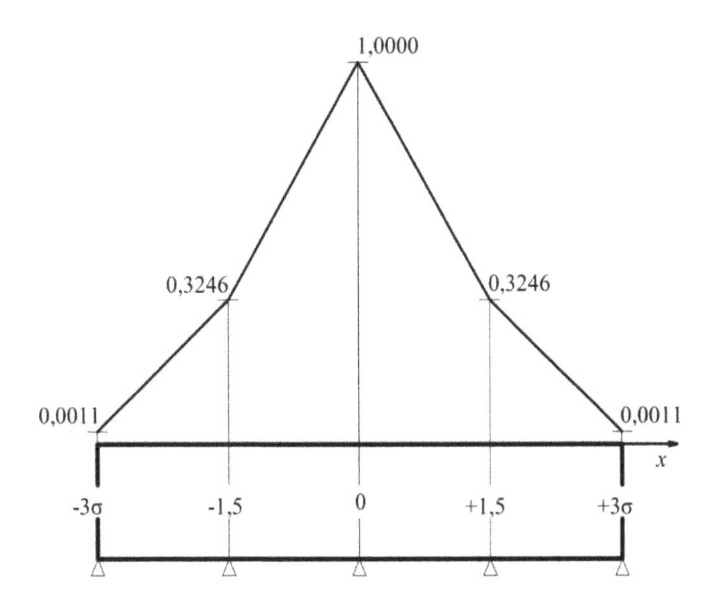

Figure 7. Five-term Gaussian function of membership (Θ = 5).

It is important to note that though fig. 6 in appearance resembles the so-called MF triangular number, but in no case should be confused with it, because of "eine grosse Kleinigkeit" (German) – zero GM value at its left and right edges.

Logical summands of FM (37) – (39) are the GM of terms provided with subscripts or superscripts, except the modal term, which GM always equals to 1. These subscripts and superscripts indicate the number of root-mean-square deviations σ along PI x axis of current terms from the modal term, with relevant sign. Positive deviations are contained in superscripts, negative deviations – in subscripts.

For the majority of practical measurements, it is quite sufficient to evaluate the combined limiting measurement error κ_r using three-term FM (37). Combined limiting spread of PI x is most conveniently represented by five-term FM (38) and by seven-term FM (39).

Let us assume that the dimension of the component is checked by a checking measurement system employing a double-limit electric contact sensor, and has FM (37) for the limiting spread of sensor contacts triggering.

$$\mathrm{v}_{sensor} = \left\langle 0.01_{-1} + 1.00 + 0.01^{+1} \right\rangle, \tag{44}$$

figure 8 a, where values −1,0 μm of subscript and +1,0 μm of superscript of GM 0,01 for two utmost terms correspond to combined limiting error ±1 μm of sensor contacts triggering.

Let us assume a priori, in the first approximation, that the spread of the dimension of a component corresponds to FM (39) in the form

$$\mathbf{v}_{comp} = \left\langle 0.01_{-3} + 0.14_{-2} + 0.61_{-1} + 1.00 + 0.61^{+1} + 0.14^{+2} + 0.01^{+3} \right\rangle \tag{45}$$

graphically presented in fig. 8 b.

As seen from FM (39), the width of its carrier in the units of measurement of subscripts and superscripts equals to 6 μm. GM values in formulas (40) and (41) are given with accuracy of two digits after decimal point, which is practically sufficient for performing logical operations (algebraic operations using GM values will not be given here at all).

As a result of this, FM (41) is "fuzzified", creating the combined FM determined by MF summing shown in figure 8.

Then let us proceed with check by measurement. From MF point of view, check operation means alignment of the left ($x_{\ulcorner}$) or, as the case may be, right ($x_{\urcorner}$) thresholds – limits of tolerance zone of component dimension, i.e. FM carrier (38), with the appropriate position of sensor contacts triggering adjusted for each of these thresholds. This alignment causes triggering of sensor contacts, in this case – at the low limit of sensor adjustment, introducing into FM (38) the check error characterized by FM (39). As the result, FM (38) is "fuzzified",

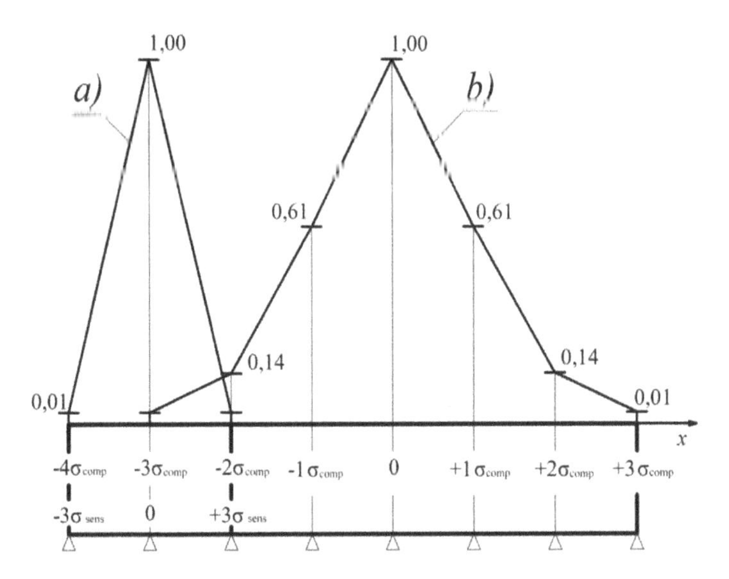

Figure 8. Mathematically fuzzy relationships during check by measurement of component dimensions using electrical contact sensor at the lower limit of tolerance zone. *a* i *b* – functions of appurtenance of electric contact check errors and controlled component dimensions, respectively.

creating the combined FM determined by MF summing shown in figure 8.

Eventually, we get the required sum

$$\left\langle 0{,}01_{-4} + 0{,}01_{-3} + 0{,}14_{-2} + 0{,}61_{-1} + 1{,}00 + 0{,}61^{+1} + 0{,}14^{+2} + 0{,}01^{+3} + 0{,}01^{+4} \right\rangle, \tag{46}$$

which is the seven-term FM (39),"fuzzified" by two terms up to nine-term FM.

This leads to the following conclusions related to quality check by measurement:

1. Adjustment of triggering of any threshold checking device to one of the limits of the specified tolerance zone of PI x of the product causes additional error ω_{sensor}, located symmetrically to the left and to the right of this zone as $\omega_{sensor/2}$ with MF normalized GM η, which is not over 0,01 (more precisely, 0,0110) for a priori assumed Gaussian FM;
2. If PI x of a product is given as a functional or technological threshold, then the error ω_{sensor} introduced by threshold checking device is located symmetrically to the left and to the right from this threshold, with the same MF indices of precision as for the tolerance zone mentioned above;
3. Manufacturing of a product which quality corresponds to PI x specified by some or other method may be guaranteed by symmetrical respective narrowing of its tolerance zone.

4. In order to increase the accuracy of the results of checking PI of the product $\omega_{sensor/2}$ at the left side and at the right side, or by the same displacement to the right and to the left of the left threshold $x_{\ulcorner}$ or right threshold $x_{\urcorner}$ specified instead of it, it is necessary to reduce the error ω_{sensor} to reasonable technical-economic limits, while MF normalized GM shall be not over 0.01.

Author details

Andrey Rostovtsev

Bauman Moscow State Technical University, Russia

References

[1] Lichtenberg, H., & Kuper, B. (1975). Anwendung von Bearbeitungsfolgegraphen in der technologischen Fertigungsvorbereitung.-Wissenschaftliche Zeitschrift der Technischen Hochschule Otto von Guericke. Magdeburg B.19, H.4.

[2] Rostovtsev, A. M. (1981). Proceedings of the 5th Leningrad conference on interchangeability and accuracy of parts made of plastics. [in Russian] Leningrad: LDNTP , 67-73.

[3] Lymzin, V. N., & Rostovtsev, A. M. (1983). Analysis of Technologic Possibilities of the New Principle for Manufacturing of Aggregates. [in Russian] "Mashinovedenie" (Machine Science) (5), 56-63.

[4] Kopin, V. A., Makarov, V. L., & Rostovtsev, A. M. (1988). Processing Plastic Components [in Russian], Moscow, Khimiya 176 p.

[5] Rostovtsev, A. (2011). Mathematically Fuzzy Approach to Quality Control.- Monography "Application and Experiences of Quality Control", Riyeka (Croatia), InTech publ., , 297-314.

[6] Rostovtsev, A. M. (2011). Measurement Errors in Formation of Product Properties. [in Russian] «Mir izmereniy» (World of measurements) (9), 52-53.

[7] Avduevskiy, V. S., Yu, A., Shilinskiy, I. F., Obraztsov, et., & al, . (1985). Scientific Basics of Advanced Engineering and Technology. Edited by V.N. Lymzin [in Russian] Moscow, Mashinostroyenie 376 p.

[8] Asai, K., & Sugeno, Terano. K. (eds. Applied Fuzzy Systems. [Translated]

[9] Matsievsky, S. V. (1993). Fuzzy Sets: Educational aid. [in Russian]- Kaliningrad: Publishing House of KGU, 2004, 176 p from Japanese into Russian] Moscow,- Mir

[10] RostovtsevA.M.,(2011). Quality Check by Measurement from the Point of View of Mathematical Fuzziness. [in Russian] Proceedings of the 11th scientific and technical conference «State and Problems of Measurements». Moscow State Technical University n.a. N.E. Bauman, 26-28 of April, , 112-114.

Chapter 5

Accreditation of Biomedical Calibration Measurements in Turkey

Mana Sezdi

Additional information is available at the end of the chapter

1. Introduction

Biomedical calibration measurement is the measurement of the accuracy of the medical device or the medical system by using the standard measurement system whose accuracy is known, and is the determination and the record of the deviations. In shortly, by the biomedical calibration measurements, it is established whether the medical devices are appropriate to the international standards or not, and the problems are also determined if the device is not adequate to the international standards (Sezdi, 2012).

Biomedical calibration measurement is different from other industrial calibration studies. Measurements are generally performed where the medical device that will be tested, is used in hospital. Only some medical devices, for example pipettes, thermometers are tested in laboratory environment.

Accreditation is the appraising of a measurement service in according to the international technical criterias, is the acception of its qualification and the controlling of it regularly. For an enterprise, being accredited is a reputable status. It shows that the enterprise has a quality management system and performs the requirements of the implemented standards. The enterprices are periodically recontrolled by an accreditation agency to protect the status and to continue fulfilling of the requirements of the business standards. The controls create the most important quality assurance of the businesses that take service from these laboratories.

In many countries, from Brazilia to China, there are accreditation studies (Boldyrev et al., 2004; Boschung et al., 2001; Iglicki et al., 2006; Kartha et al., 2003; Alexander et al., 2008; Goff et al., 2009; McGrowder et al., 2010). In Turkey, the studies of accreditation is controlled by Turkish Accreditation Agency (TURKAK). If the list of the accredited laboratory is investigated from the web site of TURKAK, it is seen that there are approximately 14 accredited enterprises that give services in biomedical calibration measurements (TURKAK website). But these are not in a single accredited enterprise type. While some of them are accepted as testing laboratories, some of them are accepted as calibration laboratories, the others are accepted as inspection bodies.

The standard used in the accreditation of testing laboratories and calibration laboratories is TS EN ISO/IEC 17025:2005. ISO 17025 contains the quality management system of the testing and calibration laboratory. It examines all work flows, organization structure and technical suffiency. The standard used in the accreditation of inspection bodies is TS EN ISO/IEC 17020:2004 (ISO IEC 17025, 2005; ISO IEC 17020, 2004).

There is not yet a specific study about the medical accreditaton in TURKAK. If hospitals demand the medical accreditation during they take the medical calibration service, they must work with the accredited laboratory in according to their measured medical device or system. It can be a medical device, radiological system or only a parameter such as temperature, mass...etc. There is a confusion about which accreditation studies should preferred for which medical devices. Is the accreditation certificate about non-medical parameters sufficient technically for biomedical calibration? In other words, is testing of a defibrilator by the mass accreditation or testing of an anesthetic machine by the temperature accreditation, ethical?

There may be many parameters that must be considered during the biomedical calibration measurements of any medical device. For example, testing of a ventilator contains flow, pressure and volume parameters. If a sufficieny is wanted, sufficiency about three parameters must be wanted seperately. In addition to this, the personnel who will perform the measurement, must be professional. The biomedical calibration needs the specialization of the biomedical personnel. It brings many problems that the biomedical calibration is performed by the non-educated personnel about biomedical and that the industrial accreditation is accepted as sufficient. Particularly, inattentive studies, in operation rooms and intensive care rooms, causes many unexpected problems.

The important point that attracts the attention in this study is that the hospitals take the inadequate services if they don't investigate the accreditation content. If the content of the accreditation studies is known, the customer will be knowledgeable about which accreditation should be preferred for which medical device or medical system.

2. Accreditation

Accreditation is a quality infrastructure tool which supports the credibility and value of the work carried out by conformity assessment bodies. Accreditation provides formal recognition that an organisation is meeting internationally accepted standards of quality, performance, technical expertise, and competence.

A product or service accompanied by a conformity attestation delivered by an accredited conformity assessment body inspires trust as to the compliance with applicable specified requirements. Thereby accreditation favours the elimination of technical barriers to trade. Accreditation provides a global acceptance of the services and establishs a confidence for the quality.

The trusting mechanism between accreditation bodies is constructed on the multi literal agreements at the international and regional accreditation body organisations, like IAF (International Accreditation Forum), ILAC (International Laboratory Accreditation Cooperation), EA (Europen Cooperation for Accreditation), etc.

Turkish Accreditation Agency (TURKAK) started to provide accrediation services in 2001 and became a cooperator of Europian Cooperation for Accreditation (EA) for all available accreditation schemes at 2008. Currently TURKAK is a full member of EA, IAF and ILAC. It serves as international accreditation agency.

Accreditation is beneficial to the accredited body itself, to Government and to users of accredited bodies.

Accredited bodies have benefits as below:

1. the laboratories are controlled by independent conformity assessment bodies and they meet international standards for competence,
2. an effective marketing tool is provided,
3. the measurements are demonstrated as traceble in according to the national or international standards,

Accredited service provides benefits for customers:

1. assurance that tests are performed by using calibrated equipment by personnel with the right level of expertise,
2. assurance that calibration or test devices are controlled and traced periodically in according to the international standards,
3. elimination of technical barriers to trade,
4. addition of credibility to the test results by accredited conformity assessment bodies,

Generally, accreditation applications are classified as 4 items.

- Accreditation of testing, calibration and medical laboratories,
- accreditation of product, service or inspection,
- accreditation of certification of management systems, and
- accreditation of personal certification bodies.

In laboratory and inspection accreditation, high respectability both at the national and international level as an indicator of technical competence is essential. Laboratory and inspection accreditation aim to give services accurate and reliable testing, analysis or calibration measurements. Laboratory accreditation ensures the official recognition of laboratory competence and offers an easy method to customers in determining and choosing reliable testing, analysis and calibration services.

The process of laboratory accreditation is regulated and standardized according to the international standards. Reports and certificates issued by accredited laboratories are internationally accepted. While the standard for testing and calibration laboratories is ISO IEC 17025:2005, the standard for inspection bodies is ISO IEC 17020:2004.

Accreditation activities of certification bodies of management system provide quality of certification of management system. Accreditation services in this field is generally given for ISO 9001:2008 certification, ISO 14001:2004 certification, ISO 22000:2005 certification, ISO 27001:2005 certification and ISO 13485:2003 certification. For this type of accreditation, ISO/IEC 17021:2011 standard is used (ISO/IEC 17021, 2011).

Accreditation of personal certification bodies that certificate the personnel making conformity assessments to make their activities in accordance with specified national and international standards, is provided by using the standard of ISO/IEC 17024:2003 (ISO/IEC 17024, 2003).

Accreditation bodies use accreditation mark or logo over their certificates or reports that contain their measurement/test results. But, such logo or marks must be used only over the certificates or reports including accredited facilities. TURKAK also provides accreditation symbol to be used in the output documents to be issued for the accredited services. It contains information about the accreditation field, accreditation standard and unique number of the accredited body, the accreditation number. The logo used by TURKAK can be seen in figure 1.

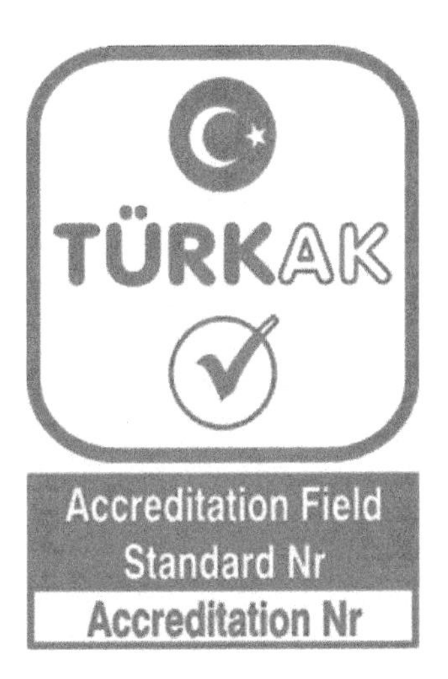

Figure 1. The accreditation logo used by TURKAK (TURKAK website).

2.1. Proficiency Testing & Interlaboratory Comparisons

For accreditation studies, the quality assurance of the test results is obtained by interlaboratory comparisons and proficiency testing (PT) (Bode, 2008; Kubota et al., 2008; Kopler et al., 2005). The interlaboratory comparisons and proficiency testing bring significant benefits to laboratories.

Proficiency Testing provides the infrastructure for a laboratory to monitor and improve the quality of its routine measurements (fig. 2). Proficiency Testing is the only quality measure which is specifically concerned with a laboratory's outputs. Proficiency Testing gives a possibility to identify any problems caused from other aspects of its quality system, such as staff training and method validation.

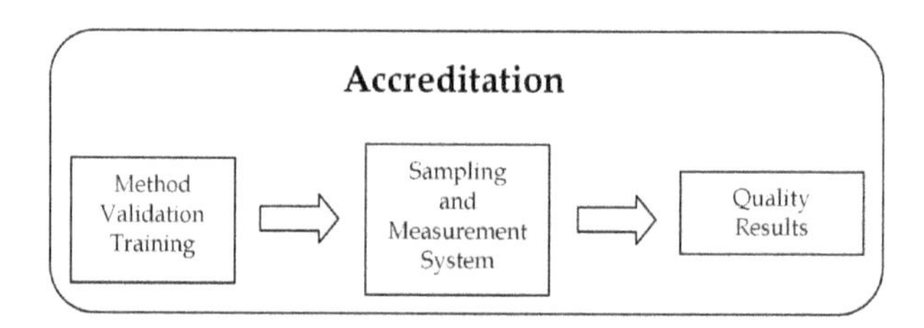

Figure 2. The factors in accreditation process.

Proficiency Testing is treated as important performance criteria regarding the evaluation of the technical competence of the laboratories. Laboratories that will be accredited should participate to Proficiency Testing programme or/and interlaboratory comparison for the main and sub disciplines they demand for accreditation and should submit satisfactory results according to defined criterias.

Proficiency Testing providers demonstrate the quality of their Proficiency Testing programmes. There are two important international guides to which Proficiency Testing providers can demonstrate the quality of their Proficiency Testing programmes:

1. ISO/IEC 17043: Conformity assessment - General requirements for proficiency testing (ISO/IEC 17043, 2007)
2. ILAC G13: Guidelines for the Requirements for the Competence of Providers of Proficiency Testing Schemes (ILAC G13, 2007)

The basic of the ISO/IEC 17043 is the ISO/IEC Guide 43. For several years, this document has provided several guidance on the development and operation laboratory proficiency testing for a relatively new field of activity. It contained very basic guidance and little attention to the use of the outcomes by laboratory accreditation bodies (Tholen, 2007).

Guide 43 have provided guidance in 5 areas (ISO Guide 43, 1997). They are;

- to distinguish between use of interlaboratory comparisons for Proficiency Testing and for other purposes (introduction to Part 1)

- the development and operation of Proficiency Testing schemes (Part 1)
- the selection and the use of schemes by laboratory accreditation bodies (Part 2)
- guidance on statistical methods (Annex A) and
- guidelines for development of a quality manual for the operation of Proficiency Testing schemes (Annex B)

The statistical annex led to the development of ILAC Guide 13. ILAC G13 contains the technical guidelines from Guide 43-1 expressed as requirements and includes the quality management system requirements from ISO/IEC Guide 25. Since G13 has management system requirements that are consistent with ISO/IEC 17025, Proficiency Testing providers accredited to this document are considered to be in conformity with the requirements of ISO 9001:2000 (Tholen, 2007). The standard ISO/IEC 17043 describes the criteria concerning the quality to be respected when developing proficiency tests and the use that can be made of these tests by the accreditation bodies. ILAC-G13 is useful to organizers for competence (Fraville et al., 2010).

The Proficiency Testing programmes of many Proficiency Testing providers around the world are now accredited by their national accreditation bodies, normally against the above documents. However, not all countries are ready to accredit Proficiency Testing providers, and not all Proficiency Testing providers wish to be accredited.

Proficiency Testing programmes are operated by a variety of organizations within Europe and the rest of the world. Many Proficiency Testing programmes are international. There is a database of available Proficiency Testing programmes. In selecting the most appropriate Proficiency Testing it is important to consider a number of issues in order to judge its suitability for your purpose (ISO Guide 34, 2000; ISO Guide 43, 1997).

3. Accreditation Standards

The accreditation standards used in biomedical calibration measurements can be classified into 2 groups. TS EN ISO / IEC 17025 and TS EN ISO / IEC 17020. While the standard of 17025 is used for the accreditation of testing and calibration laboratories, the standard of 17020 is used for the accreditation of inspection bodies.

The laboratory accreditation standards should not be confused with ISO 9001 standard. ISO 9001 is widely used in the assessment of the quality systems of production and service organizations. Certification of organizations according to the ISO 9001 system expresses the compliance of that organization's quality system with this standard (ISO 9001). When certifying laboratories according to ISO 9001, this certification makes no statement on the technical competence of laboratories. From this point, the certificate's power to convince the market and prospects of laboratories is quiet insufficient.

3.1. The standard of TS EN ISO / IEC 17025

ISO IEC 17025, entitled "General Requirements for the Competence of Testing and Calibration Laboratories", is an international standard describing the general requirements to meet for the recognition of that a laboratory is competent to perform specific tests (ISO IEC 17025; 2005). This international standard is used to develop the quality, management and technical systems of laboratories (Abdel-Fatah, 2010; Glavic-Cindro et al., 2006; Brantner et al., 2011; Zapata-Garcia et al., 2007; Jerone et al., 2008). Technical requirements are updated to include the addition of formal personnel training plans and detailed records, method development and validation procedures, measurement of method uncertainty, and a defined equipment calibration and maintenance program (Honsa et al., 2003). ISO 17025 certification can be applied to all organizations that give services of testing or calibration. These organizations are the first-party, second-party and third-party laboratories.

First–party Laboratories: Manufacturer Laboratories, Second-party Laboratories: Customer Laboratories, Third-party Laboratories: Independent Laboratories.

This standard can be applied to all laboratories regardless of the scope of test or calibration activities and the number of personnel.

If testing and calibration laboratories comply with the requirements of this standard, a quality management system to meet the principles of ISO 9001 will be also applied. There is a cross-match among TS EN ISO 17025 standard and ISO 9001. TS EN ISO 17025 standard covers technical competence requirements, not covered by ISO 9001.

3.1.1. The content of the standard of TS EN ISO / IEC 17025

TS EN ISO 17025 standard is assessed in two main categories. The standard of TS EN ISO IEC 17025 contains both the management and technical requirements. In standard, 4th item describes the management system and 5th item describes the technical activities. The content of 17025 standard is as follows:

0 Introduction

1 Scope

2 Cited in standards and / or documents

3 Terms and definitions

4 Management requirements

4.1 Organization

4.2 Management system

4.3 Document control

4.4 Review of requests, tenders and contracts

4.5 Subcontracting of tests and calibrations

4.6 Purchasing of service and materials

4.7 Customer service 4.8 Complaints

4.8 Complaints

4.9 Control of nonconforming testing and / or calibration work

4.10 Improvement

4.11 Corrective action

4.12 Preventive action

4.13 Control of records

4.14 Internal controls

4.15 Management reviews

5 Technical requirements

5.1 General

5.2 Personnel

5.3 Accommodation and environmental conditions

5.4 Test and calibration methods and method validation

5.5 Devices

5.6 Measurement traceability

5.7 Sampling

5.8 Calibration procedures

5.9 Assuring the quality of test and calibration results

5.10 Reporting of the results

The laboratory must be an institution that can be held legally responsible. Laboratory management system must consist of facilities in fixed laboratory and temporary or mobile facilities that are linked to the laboratory.

3.2. The standard of TS EN ISO / IEC 17020

ISO 17020, entitled "General Criteria for the Operation of Various Types of Bodies Performing Inspection", is an internationally recognized standard for the competence of inspection bodies. Inspection parameters may include such aspects as the quantity, quality, safety, suitability, facilities or systems (ISO IEC 17020; 2004).

There are 3 types of inspection organizations. They are:

Type A: Inspection body must be independent. Both the inspection organization and its personnel must not be related to the inspected materials. They must not be the material's designers, manufacturers, suppliers, installers, purchasers, owners or operators.

Type B: Inspection services should be given to the organization that consists of the inspection body. Type B bodies can not service to other organizations.

Type C: This type of bodies give services to both the organization that consists of the inspection body and other organizations.

TS EN ISO 17020 standard can be applied regardless of the scope of inspection activities in the company. TS EN ISO 17020 certification can be given all kinds of inspection bodies that are willing to give service in accordance with this standard.

3.2.1. The content of the standard of TS EN ISO / IEC 17020

In the standard of TS EN ISO IEC 17020, the technical requirements are the main aspect. TS EN ISO 17020 standard consists of 16 items. They are:

0 Introduction

1 Scope

2 Definitions

3 Administrative Rules

4 Independence, impartiality and integrity

5 Privacy

6 Organization and management

7 Quality System

8 Personnel

9 Equipment

10 Inspection methods and procedures

11 Samples and materials to be inspected

12 Records

13 Inspection reports and inspection certificates

14 The use of subcontractors

15 Complaints and appeals

16 Co-operation

4. Accreditation Types

As it was mentioned earlier, there are 3 accreditation types for biomedical calibration measurements. They are:

- Calibration laboratories

- Testing laboratories
- Inspection bodies

4.1 Calibration Laboratories

A calibration laboratory is a laboratory that performs test, calibration and repair of measuring instruments. The calibration of equipment is achieved by means of a direct comparison against measurement standards or certified reference materials. These standards are also regularly calibrated themselves, in comparison with another standard of lower uncertainty.

Measurement Parameter	Example Measurement Range	Measurement Condition	Example Measurement Uncertainty	Method Standard
Pressure	0 - 70 bar	Air	0,2 %	Euramet CG-17 / v.01
	70 - 700 bar	Hydraulic	0,2 %	
Temperature distribution of controlled volume	-40 +200 °C	In controlled volume (oven, incubator, freezer....)	0,68 °C	Euramet CG-13 / v.01
Scales (non automatic)	0 – 600 gr	E2 class mass	$2\ 10^{-6}$	Euramet CG-18 / v.03
	0 – 10 kg	F1 class mass	$1\ 10^{-5}$	
	0 – 150 kg	M1 class mass	$1\ 10^{-4}$	
	0 – 1000 kg	M1-M2 mass	$2\ 10^{-4}$	
Temperature of glass thermometer	0 – 60 °C	Water bath	0,72 °C	Measurement in laboratory by using comparison method
	60 – 150 °C	Dry block oil bath	0,74 °C	
Volume Piston pipettes	50 – 100 µl	in laboratory	0,100 µl	TS ISO 4787 TS EN ISO 8655-2 TS EN ISO 8655-6
	200 µl		0,158 µl	
	500 µl		0,315 µl	
	1 ml		0,452 µl	
	2 ml		1,209 µl	
	5 ml		2,851 µl	
	10 ml		5,991 µl	
Temperature meters with display	0 – 250 °C	Ice bath and dry block oven	0,56 °C	Measurement in laboratory by using comparison method
	250 – 600 °C		0,82 °C	
Moisture	20% - 70% RH	Humidity cabinet	1,4% RH	Measurement in laboratory by using comparison method
	70% - 90% RH		2,2% RH	

Table 1. The content of accreditation studies of calibration laboratories.

Calibration laboratories give services to all industry, textile, paint, food or health care etc. The company's working area is not important. The parameter to be measured is essential. For example, the mass for the weighing of food, rotational speed of the paint mixing device, hardness of the material used in manufacturing, the temperature of refrigerators used for drug store. The parameters are measured and a calibration certificate is prepared.

The biomedical measurements in calibration laboratories are also performed generally as parameter measurements. The parameters can be classified as electrical parameters, pressure-vacuum parameters, temperature-humidity parameters, mass-volume parameters. An example study for accreditation of calibration laboratories can be seen in Table 1.

The accreditation of calibration measurements is carried out via parameter measurements. Unlike other types of accreditation studies, parameter measurement is accredited for calibration laboratory. As of today, ISO IEC 17025 is taken as the basis for laboratory accreditation purposes. This standard is recognized worldwide. The requirements of this standard are provided for the general requirements on a laboratory's quality management system and technical competence. Laboratories accredited according to ISO IEC 17025 are re-evaluated periodically by the accreditation body and decision is made for the maintenance of accreditation based on results obtained.

Laboratories intending to maintain accreditation are required to participate inter-laboratory comparison and proficiency testing programs on their scope of accreditation and achieve successful results.

4.2. Testing Laboratories

The biomedical measurements in testing laboratories are performed on the basis of the medical device. The test procedures are prepared to test all parameters in the medical device. Defibrillators, ventilators...etc. are tested completely to measure all parameters in it. If there are many parameters in a device such as ECG parameters (electrical), blood pressure parameters (pressure), body temperature parameters (temperature), they are measured in according to the measurement procedures in the place of where medical device works and a certificate is prepared.

In Turkey, the standard of 17025 is applied to testing laboratories for the medical devices. The content of the accreditation studies of testing laboratories can be seen in Table 2 and Table 3.

Device Under Test	Testing Name	Testing Method - Standard
Electrical Safety Tests for all Electrical Biomedical Devices	Earth resistance	TS EN 60601-1 (item 8.7)
	Chassis leakage current	TS EN 60601-1 (item 8.7)
	Patient leakage current	TS EN 60601-1 (item 8.7)
	Patient auxiliary leakage current	TS EN 60601-1 (item 8.7)

Device Under Test	Testing Name	Testing Method - Standard
	Applied part leakage current	TS EN 60601-1 (item 8.7)
	[illegible]	[illegible]
	DC chassis voltage	TS EN 60601-1 (item 8.9)
	Mains voltage	TS EN 60601-1 (item 8)
	Device current	TS EN 60601-1 (item 8)
Performance-Safety Tests for Defibrillators	ECG pulse test	TS EN 60601-2-27 (item 50.102.15)
	ECG amplitude test	TS EN 60601-2-27 (item 50.102.15)
	ECG frequency test	TS EN 60601-2-27 (item 50.102.8)
	ECG arythmia test	TS EN 60601-2-27 (item 56.8)
	Energy test	TS EN 60601-2-4 (item 50)
	Charge time test	TS EN 60601-2-4 (item 101)
	Synchronized discharge test	TS EN 60601-2-4 (item 104)
Performance-Safety Tests for Electrosurgical Units	Power distribution test	TS EN 60601-2-2 (item 50.1)
	HF leak test	TS EN 60601-2-2 (item 19.3.101)
	REM alarm test	TS EN 60601-2-2 (item 52)
Performance-Safety Tests for Pulse Oximeter (sPO2)	sPO2 performans test	TS EN ISO 9919 (item 50.101)
	ECG pulse test	TS EN 60601-2-27 (item 50.102.15)
	sPO2 alarm test	TS EN ISO 9919 (item 104)
Performance-Safety Tests for Electrocardiography (ECG)	ECG pulse test	TS EN 60601-2-27 (item 50.102.15)
	ECG amplitude test	TS EN 60601-2-27 (item 50.102.15)
	ECG frequency test	TS EN 60601-2-27 (item 50.102.8)
	ECG arythmia test	TS EN 60601-2-27 (item 56.8)
	ECG ST test	TS EN 60601-2-27 (item 50.102.15)
	ECG printer test	TS EN 60601-2-27 (item 50.102.16)
Performance-Safety Tests for Noninvasive Blood Pressure Monitor (NIBP)	NIBP performans test	TS EN 60601-2-30 (item 50.2)
	NIBP cuff pressure test	TS EN 60601-2-30 (item 22.4.1)
	NIBP cuff leakage test	TS EN 60601-2-30 (item 50.2)
	NIBP alarm test	TS EN 60601-2-30 (item 51.103)
Performance-Safety Tests for Aspirators	Vacuum test	TS EN ISO 10079-1
	Accuracy test	TS EN ISO 10079-1
	Flow test	TS EN ISO 10079-1

Table 2. The content of accreditation studies of testing laboratories.

Device Under Test	Testing Name	Testing Method - Standard
Performance-Safety Tests for Infusion Pumps	Air control test	TS EN 60601-1-24 (item 51-104)
	Flow accuracy test	TS EN 60601-1-24 (item 50-103)
	Congestion performance test	TS EN 60601-1-24 (item 2-122)
	Alarm test	TS EN 60601-1-24 (item 51-106)
Performance-Safety Tests for Aspirators	Vacuum test	TS EN ISO 10079-1
	Accuracy test	TS EN ISO 10079-1
	Flow test	TS EN ISO 10079-1
Performance-Safety Tests for Shymphonometers	System leak test	TS EN 1060
	Manometer test	TS EN 1060
	Accuracy test	TS EN 1060
Performance-Safety Tests for Patient Monitor	ECG pulse test	TS EN 60601-2-27 (item 50.102.15)
	ECG amplitude test	TS EN 60601-2-27 (item 50.102.15)
	ECG frequency test	TS EN 60601-2-27 (item 50.102.8)
	ECG arythmia test	TS EN 60601-2-27 (item 56.8)
	ECG ST test	TS EN 60601-2-27 (item 50.102.15)
	ECG printer test	TS EN 60601-2-27 (item 50.102.16)
	Pacemaker test	TS EN 60601-2-27 (item 50.102.12)
	ECG alarm test	TS EN 60601-2-27 (item 51.102)
	Breath performance test	TS EN 60601-2-27 (item 50.102.8)
	Breath alarm test	TS EN 60601-2-27 (item 51.102)
	NIBP performans test	TS EN 60601-2-30 (item 50.2)
	NIBP cuff pressure test	TS EN 60601-2-30 (item 22.4.1)
	NIBP cuff leakage test	TS EN 60601-2-30 (item 50.2)
	NIBP alarm test	TS EN 60601-2-30 (item 51.103)
	IBP static pressure test	TS EN 60601-2-34 (item 51.102)
	IBP dynamic pressure	TS EN 60601-2-34 (item 51.102)
	IBP alarm test	TS EN 60601-2-34 (item 51.203.1)
	sPO2 performans test	TS EN ISO 9919 (item 50.101)
	sPO2 alarm test	TS EN ISO 9919 (item 104)

Table 3. The content of accreditation studies of testing laboratories (continued).

4.3. Inspection Bodies

Inspection bodies which applied for accreditation must accomplish the requirements of standard ISO IEC 17020:2004. Inspection means investigation of the product design, product, service, process of the factory and their professional judgment based on the determination of the conformity of the general rules. Inspection bodies are conformity assessment companies. After the inspection, they transmit report to the customer, no certification. In Turkey, 17020 standard is applied for the radiography systems and clean room classification. The content of the accreditation studies of inspection bodies can be seen in Table 4.

Medical Device	Inspection Type	Standard
CONVENTIONAL RADIOGRAPHY	kVp	IPEM Report No 32, European Commission Radiation Protection No 91
	Exposure time	IPEM Report No 32, European Commission Radiation Protection No 91
	Exposure repeatability and linearity	IPEM Report No 32, AAPM Report No 74, European Commission Radiation Protection No 91
	Tube output and stability	IPEM Report No 32, European Commission Radiation Protection No 91
	Filtration and half value layer	IPEM Report No 32, AAPM Report No 74, FDA 21 CFR 1020.30, European Commission Radiation Protection No 91
	Collimation	IPEM Report No 32, European Commission Radiation Protection No 91
	X-ray beam alignment	European Commission Radiation Protection No 91
	Focal spot size	IPEM Report No 32, European Commission Radiation Protection No 91
	Automatic exposure control	IPEM Report No 32, European Commission Radiation Protection No 91
	Grid adjustment	European Commission Radiation Protection No 91 AAPM Report No 74
	Leakage radiation	European Commission Radiation Protection No 91 FDA 21 CFR 1020.30
INTRA-ORAL and	kVp	European Commission Radiation Protection No 91 IPEM Report No 91

Medical Device	Inspection Type	Standard
PANORAMIC CONVENTIONAL DENTAL RADIOGRAPHY	Exposure time	European Commission Radiation Protection No 91 IPEM Report No 91
	Tube output	European Commission Radiation Protection No 91
	Patient entrance dose	IPEM Report N:91, European Commission Radiation Protection N 162
	Filtration and half value layer	European Commission Radiation Protection No 91 FDA 21 CFR 1020.30
	X-ray beam size	European Commission Radiation Protection No 91 IPEM Report No 91
	Patient focus distance	European Commission Radiation Protection No 91
	Image repeatability	IPEM Report No 91
CONVENTIONAL MAMMOGRAPHY	Focus film distance	European Commission European Guidelines for Quality in Breast Cancer Screening and Diagnosis
	Tissue thickness sensor	IPEM Report 89
	Compression force	European Commission Radiation Protection No 91,
	kVp accuracy and repeatability	European Commission European Guidelines for Quality in Breast Cancer Screening and Diagnosis, European Commission Radiation Protection No 91, ACR Mammography QC Manual
	Tube output, tube output speed and repeatability	European Commission European Guidelines for Quality in Breast Cancer Screening and Diagnosis, European Commission Radiation Protection No 91 IPSM Report N59, ACR Mammography QC Manual, IPEM Report No 89
	Tube output-mAs	IPEM Report No 91, IPEM Report No 89
	Filtration and half value layer	European Commission European Guidelines for Quality in Breast Cancer Screening and Diagnosis, IPEM Report 89, ACR Mammography QC Manual
	Mean glandular tissue dose	European Commission European Guidelines for Quality in Breast Cancer Screening and Diagnosis, ACR Mammography QC Manual

Medical Device	Inspection Type	Standard
	Image contrast and high [illegible]	European Commission European Guidelines for Quality in Breast Cancer Screening and Diagnosis, European Commission Radiation Protection No 91 and 162, ACR Mammography QC Mn
	Collimation, Grid factor and determination of grid errors	European Commission European Guidelines for Quality in Breast Cancer Screening and Diagnosis, IPEM Report 89, European Commission Radiation Protection 91, ACR Mammo QC Manual
	Image homogeneity and assessment of artifacts	European Commission European Guidelines for Quality in Breast Cancer Screening and Diagnosis, IPEM Report 89, ACR Mammography QC Manual
	Leakage radiation	European Commission European Guidelines for Quality in Breast Cancer Screening and Diagnosis
DIGITAL (FLAT PANEL) and CONVENTIONAL IMAGE AMPLIFIED FLOROSCOPY (DSA ANJIO, CARDIAC, C ARM MOBIL)	kVp	IPEM Report No 32, IPEM Report No 91, European Commission Radiation Protection No 91, AAPM Report No 74
	Filtration and half value layer	IPEM Report No 32, IPEM Report No 91, IPEM Report No 32, European Commission Radiation Protection No 91, AAPM Report No 74
	Tube Output	IPEM Report No 32, AAPM Report N:70
	Maximum exposure speed	European Commission Radiation Protection No 91 and 162, IPEM Report No 32, AAPM Report No 70 - 74
	Patient entrance dose	Draft European Commission Radiation Protection No 162, AAPM Report No 70, AAPM Report No 74
	Image amplified entrance dose	European Commission Radiation Protection No 91 and 162, AAPM Report No 70 and 74
	Brightness control	IPEM Report N:32, AAPM Report No 70
	Gray scale	IPEM Report No 32
	Image artifacts	IPEM Report No 32
	Compliance of areas (exposured-displayed)	European Commission Radiation Protection No 91, IPEM Report No 32

Medical Device	Inspection Type	Standard
	High contrast and low contrast resolution	European Commission Radiation Protection No 91, IPEM Report No 32
	Contrast detail	IPEM Report No 32
FLOROSCOPY RADIOGRAPY (STOMACH TABLE)	kVp	IPEM Report No 91
	Exposure time	IPEM Report No 91 and 32, European Commission Radiation Protection No 91
	Exposure repeatability and linearity	IPEM Report No 91 and 32, European Commission Radiation Protection No 91, AAPM Report No 74
	Tube output and stability	IPEM Report No 91 and 32, European Commission Radiation Protection No 91
	Collimation	IPEM Report No 91 and 32, European Commission Radiation Protection No 91
	Gray scale	IPEM Report No 32
	High contrast and low contrast resolution	European Commission Radiation Protection No 91, Draft European Commission Radiation Protection No 162, IPEM Report No 32
	Contrast detail	IPEM Report No 32
COMPUTED TOMOGRAPHY	kVp	IPEM Report No 32,
	Half value layer test	IPEM Report No 32,
	Position of external and internal scanning lights	IPEM Report No 32, IPEM Report No 91
	Coronal and Sagittal Alignment	IPEM Report No 32, IPEM Report No 91
	The slope of gantry	AAPM Report No 39
	Table axial motion accuracy	IPEM Report No 32, IPEM Report No 91, IEC 61223-2-6
	Table helical motion accuracy	IPEM Report No 32, IPEM Report No 91, IEC 61223-2-6
	Table distance sensor	IPEM Report No 32, IPEM Report No 91
	Computed tomography dose index (CTDI)	IPEM Report No 32, EC EUR 16262
	Tube output (CTDI Air) and linearity	IPEM Report No 32
	Slice thickness	IPEM Report No 32, IEC 61223-2-6

Medical Device	Inspection Type	Standard
	CT number linearity	IPEM Report No 32, IPEM Report No 91
	Highcontrastresolution	IPEM Report N.32 and 91, IEC 61223-2-6
	Low contrast resolution	IPEM Report No 32
	Noise measurement	NCRPM Report No 99, IPEM Report No 32 and 91
	CT number uniformity	IPEM Report N:32 and 91, IEC 61223-2-6
ULTRASOUND DEVICE	Image homogeneity	AAPM Report of Task Group No 1
	Image depth	AAPM Report of Task Group No 1
	Distance accuracy	AAPM Report of Task Group No 1
	Axial resolution	AAPM Report of Task Group No 1
	Lateral resolution	AAPM Report of Task Group No 1
	Dead zone	AAPM Report of Task Group No 1
	Cyst diameter	AAPM Report of Task Group No 1
NEGATOSKOP and VIEWING ROOM	Negatoskop brigthness and levels of bright of viewing room	IPEM Report 89, IPEM Report No 32, European Commission European Guidelines for Quality in Breast Cancer Screening and Diagnosis, ACR Mammography QC Manual

Table 4. The content of accreditation studies of inspection bodies.

5. Discussion

In Turkey, accreditation studies about biomedical calibration are performed in 3 different types. Calibration laboratories, testing laboratories and inspection bodies. Normally, although the scope of their applications seems like they are nested, they are separated from each other with little detail. Inspections of radiography devices and clean rooms are performed by inspection bodies. Other medical devices except for pipettes, thermometers, humidity meters that must be measured in laboratory conditions, are tested by testing laboratories and they are accredited in according to the standard of ISO IEC 17025. In calibration laboratories, it is essential to ensure appropriate environmental conditions for measurements. Because of this, measurements that require special measuring environment are performed in calibration laboratories.

If the differences and details of accreditation studies about biomedical calibration measurements are known by the health organizations, to make the right choice in the selection of calibration laboratory, testing laboratory or inspection body is inevitable.

6. Conclusion

Quality service can be only taken from the accredited laboratories. As a matter of fact, the national and international procedures of accreditation say, "There is not an obligation. The accreditation depends on the base of voluntary." (TURKAK website).

Even if accreditation is not obligated, the expectation in medical calibration measurements is that the personnel must be professional, the calibration procedures and the test devices, calibrators must be appropriate to the international standards.

Acknowledgements

I would like to thank the co-operation of the calibration laboratories, the testing laboratories and the inspection bodies that present the content of their accreditation studies.

Author details

Mana Sezdi[1*]

Address all correspondence to: mana@istanbul.edu.tr

1 Istanbul University, Turkey

References

[1] Abdel-Fatah Hesham , T. M. (2010, January). ISO/IEC 17025 Accreditation: Between the desired gains and the reality. *Journal of Quality Assurance*, 13(1), 21-27.

[2] Alexander, B. J. R., Flynn, A. R., Gibbons, A. M., Clover, G. R. G., & Herrera, V. E. (2008). New Zealand perspective on ISO 17025 accreditation of a plant diagnostic laboratory. *Bulletin OEPP*, 38(2), 172-177.

[3] Brantner, C., Pope, R., Hannah, R., & Burans, J. (2011, July). Preparing a biological electron microscopy laboratory for ISO 17025 accreditation. *Microscopy & Microanalysis*, 17(52), 1154-1155.

[4] Bode, P. (2008, August). Role and evaluation of interlaboratory comparison results in laboratory accreditation. *AIP Conference Proceedings*, 1036(1), 29-37.

[5] Boldyrev, I. V., & Karpov, Y. A. (2004, January). Implementation of ISO/IEC 17025 standard for the accreditation of analytical laboratories in Russia. *Accreditation and Quality Assurance*, 9(1-2), 99-105.

[6] Boschung, M., & Wernli, C. (2001). Accreditation of a personal dosimetry service in Switzerland. Practical experience and transition from EN450004 to ISO 17025. *Radiation Protection Dosimetry*, 96(1-3), 123-126.

[7] Fraville, L., Moulut, J. C., Grzebyk, M., & Kauffer, F. (2010). Producing samples for the organization of proficiency tests. Study of the homogeneity of replicas produced from two atmosphere generation systems. *Annual Occupational Hygiene Society*, 1-12.

[8] Glavic-Cindro, D., & Korun, M. (2006). Influence of a quality system complying with the requirements of ISO/IEC 17025 standard on the management of a gamma ray spectrometry laboratory. *Accreditation and Quality Assurance,*, 10, 609-612.

[9] Goff, T. Le., Joseph, B., & Wood, S. (2009). Development and accreditation to ISO/IEC 17025 calibration status of a melting point measurement facility for the UK. *Journal of Thermal Analysis and Calorimetry*, 96, 653-662.

[10] Honsa, J. D., & Mclntyre, D. A. (2012, February). ISO 17025: Practical benefits of implementing a quality system. *Journal of AOAC International*, 86(5), 1038-1044.

[11] Iglicki, A., Mila, M. I., Furnari, J. C., Arenillas, P., Cerutti, G., Carballido, M., Guillen, V., Araya, X., & Bianchini, R. (2006). Accreditation experience of radioisotope metrology laboratory of Argentina. *Applied Radiation and Isotopes*, 64(10-11), 1171-1173.

[12] ILAC G13. (2007). *Guidelines for the Requirements for the Competence of Providers of Proficiency Testing Schemes*, International Laboratory Accreditation Cooperation, Australia.

[13] ISO Guide 34. (2000). *General requirements for the competence of reference material providers*, International Organization for Standardization, Geneva.

[14] ISO Guide 43. (1997). *Proficiency testing by interlaboratory by comparisons- Part 1: Development and operation of proficiency testing schemes*, International Organization for Standardization, Geneva.

[15] ISO IEC 17020. (2004). *General criteria for the operation of various types of bodies performing inspection*, International Organization for Standardization, Geneva.

[16] ISO IEC 17021. (2011). *Conformity assessment- Requirements for bodies providing audit and certification of management systems*, International Organization for Standardization, Geneva.

[17] ISO IEC 17024. (2003). *Conformity assessment- General requirements for bodies operating certification of persons*, International Organization for Standardization, Geneva.

[18] ISO IEC 17025 (2005). General requirements for the competence of testing and calibration laboratories. International Organization for Standardization, Geneva, (2005)

[19] ISO IEC (17043). (2007). Conformity assessment-- General requirements for proficiency testing. International Organization for Standardization Geneva

[20] ISO 9001. (2000). *Quality management systems-requirements*, International Organization for Standardization, Geneva.

[21] Jerone, S. M., & Judge, S. M. (2008, May). Accreditation to ISO 17025:2005 for the radioactivity metrology group of the UK's national physical laboratory. *Journal of Radioanalytical and Nuclear Chemistry*, 276(2), 353-355.

[22] Kartha, K. P. S., Ghosh, P., Varshney, K. M., & Shakla, S. K. (2003, Sep). Implementation of ISO/IEC 17025 in forensic science laboratories, An Indian perspective. *Forensic Science International*, 136, 6.

[23] Kopler, K., Viladimirov, A., & Servoman, A. (2005). Interlaboratory comparison and accreditation in quality control testing of diagnostic X-ray equipment. *Radiation Protection Dosimetry*, 114, 198-200.

[24] Kubota, M., Takata, Y., Koizumi, K., Ishibashi, Y., Matsuda, R., Matsumoto, Y., Shikakume, K., Ono, A., & Sakata, M. (2008, Jun). Proficiency testing provided by the Japan Society for analytical chemistry. *Bunseki Kagaku*, 37, 393-409.

[25] Mc Growder, D., Crawford, T., Irving, R., Brown, P., & Anderson-Jacken, L. (2010, Oct). How prepared are medical and non-medical laboratories in Jamaica for accreditation? *Accreditation and Quality Assurance*, 15(10), 569-577.

[26] Sezdi, M. (2012, June). A roadmap of Biomedical Engineers and Milestones. *Medical Technology Management and Patient Safety*, InTech.

[27] Tholen, D. W. (2007, October). ISO/IEC 17043: A new international standard for proficiency testing. Romania. *The first International Proficiency Testing Conference*, 11-13.

[28] TURKAK website: http://turkak.org.tr

[29] Zapata-Garcia, D., Llaurado, M., & Rauret, G. (2007, June). Experience of implementing ISO 17025 for the accreditation of an university testing laboratory. *Accreditation and Quality Assurance*, 12(6), 317-322.

Permissions

The contributors of this book come from diverse backgrounds, making this book a truly international effort. This book will bring forth new frontiers with its revolutionizing research information and detailed analysis of the nascent developments around the world.

We would like to thank Mohammad Saber Fallah Nezhad, for lending his expertise to make the book truly unique. He has played a crucial role in the development of this book. Without his invaluable contribution this book wouldn't have been possible. He has made vital efforts to compile up to date information on the varied aspects of this subject to make this book a valuable addition to the collection of many professionals and students.

This book was conceptualized with the vision of imparting up-to-date information and advanced data in this field. To ensure the same, a matchless editorial board was set up. Every individual on the board went through rigorous rounds of assessment to prove their worth. After which they invested a large part of their time researching and compiling the most relevant data for our readers. Conferences and sessions were held from time to time between the editorial board and the contributing authors to present the data in the most comprehensible form. The editorial team has worked tirelessly to provide valuable and valid information to help people across the globe.

Every chapter published in this book has been scrutinized by our experts. Their significance has been extensively debated. The topics covered herein carry significant findings which will fuel the growth of the discipline. They may even be implemented as practical applications or may be referred to as a beginning point for another development. Chapters in this book were first published by InTech; hereby published with permission under the Creative Commons Attribution License or equivalent.

The editorial board has been involved in producing this book since its inception. They have spent rigorous hours researching and exploring the diverse topics which have resulted in the successful publishing of this book. They have passed on their knowledge of decades through this book. To expedite this challenging task, the publisher supported the team at every step. A small team of assistant editors was also appointed to further simplify the editing procedure and attain best results for the readers.

Our editorial team has been hand-picked from every corner of the world. Their multi-ethnicity adds dynamic inputs to the discussions which result in innovative outcomes. These outcomes are then further discussed with the researchers and contributors who give their valuable feedback and opinion regarding the same. The feedback is then collaborated with the researches and they are edited in a comprehensive manner to aid the understanding of the subject.

Apart from the editorial board, the designing team has also invested a significant amount of their time in understanding the subject and creating the most relevant covers. They scrutinized every image to scout for the most suitable representation of the subject and create an appropriate cover for the book.

The publishing team has been involved in this book since its early stages. They were actively engaged in every process, be it collecting the data, connecting with the contributors or procuring relevant information. The team has been an ardent support to the editorial, designing and production team. Their endless efforts to recruit the best for this project, has resulted in the accomplishment of this book. They are a veteran in the field of academics and their pool of knowledge is as vast as their experience in printing. Their expertise and guidance has proved useful at every step. Their uncompromising quality standards have made this book an exceptional effort. Their encouragement from time to time has been an inspiration for everyone.

The publisher and the editorial board hope that this book will prove to be a valuable piece of knowledge for researchers, students, practitioners and scholars across the globe.

List of Contributors

Kenneth Hubbard, Jinsheng You and Martha Shulski
High Plains Regional Climate Center, University of Nebraska, Lincoln, NE, USA

Mohammad Saber Fallah Nezhad
Assistant Professor of Industrial Engineering, Yazd University, Iran

Suzana Leitão Russo
Department of Statistic - Federal University of Sergipe, Brazil

Maria Emilia Camargo
Post-Graduate Program in Administration, University of Caxias of South, Brazil

Jonas Pedro Fabris
Fabris Industry, Brazil

Andrey Rostovtsev
Bauman Moscow State Technical University, Russia

Mana Sezdi
Istanbul University, Turkey

Printed in the USA
CPSIA information can be obtained
at www.ICGtesting.com
JSHW011809301024
72690JS00002B/4